610-7 FRE

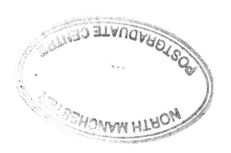

D0237219

Effective Interprofessional Education

Development, Delivery and Evaluation

Della Freeth
Marilyn Hammick
Scott Reeves
Ivan Koppel
Hugh Barr

Series editor: Hugh Barr

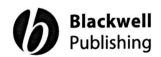

© 2005 by Blackwell Publishing Ltd

Editorial offices:
Blackwell Publishing Ltd, 9600 Garsington Road, Oxford OX4 2DQ, UK
    Tel: +44 (0)1865 776868
Blackwell Publishing Inc., 350 Main Street, Malden, MA 02148-5020, USA
    Tel: +1 781 388 8250
Blackwell Publishing Asia Pty Ltd, 550 Swanston Street, Carlton, Victoria 3053, Australia
    Tel: +61 (0)3 8359 1011

First published 2005 by Blackwell Publishing Ltd

Library of Congress Cataloging-in-Publication Data

Effective interprofessional education: development, delivery, and
        evaluation/by Della Freeth … [et al.].
        p.; cm. – (Promoting partnership for health)
        Includes bibliographical references and index.
        ISBN-13: 978-1-4051-1653-4 (hardback: alk. paper)
        ISBN-10: 1-4051-1653-6 (hardback: alk. paper)
        1. Medical education.   2. Social work education.   3. Interprofessional relations.
4. Interdisciplinary approach in education.
I. Freeth, Della. II. Series.
        [DNLM: 1. Health Occupations–education.   2. Education, Professional–methods.
3. Interdisciplinary Communication.   4. Interprofessional Relations.   5. Program Evaluation. W 18
E269 2005]
R834.E3552 2005
610′.71′1–dc22
2004030718

ISBN-13: 978-14051-1653-4
ISBN-10: 1-4051-1653-6

A catalogue record for this title is available from the British Library

Set in 10 on 12.5pt Palatino
by SPI Publisher Services, Pondicherry, India

The publisher's policy is to use permanent paper from mills that operate a sustainable forestry policy, and which has been manufactured from pulp processed using acid-free and elementary chlorine-free practices. Furthermore, the publisher ensures that the text paper and cover board used have met acceptable environmental accreditation standards.

For further information on Blackwell Publishing, visit our website:
www.blackwellpublishing.com

Contents

Contributors

Della Freeth is Reader in Education for Health Care Practice at City University, London, based in the Health Care Education Development Unit at the St Bartholomew School of Nursing and Midwifery. She is an educationalist who works alongside a wide range of health professionals, supporting the development and evaluation of educational initiatives. Her personal research interests have two overlapping foci, interprofessional collaboration and learning through simulated professional practice. She is a Board Member of CAIPE and an Associate Editor of the *Journal of Interprofessional Care*.

Marilyn Hammick is an education and research consultant, Visiting Professor of Interprofessional Education, School of Health Care Practice, Anglia Polytechnic University; Associate Editor of *Journal of Interprofessional Care*; Vice-chair of CAIPE and Consultant to Best Evidence Medical Education. Her international work includes mentoring systematic review groups and she is external evaluator to nationally funded interprofessional education projects. Marilyn was previously a Senior Lecturer, Centre for Research in Medical and Dental Education, University of Birmingham, and Reader in Interprofessional Education, Oxford Brookes University.

Scott Reeves is a Research Fellow in the Health Care Education Development Unit, St Bartholomew School of Nursing and Midwifery, City University. He is also a Senior Research Fellow at the Faculty of Health and Social Care, London South Bank University. Scott is a sociologist who collaborates with colleagues from a range of health and social care backgrounds. His work focuses on the evaluation of interprofessional education and collaboration. Scott is an Associate Editor of the *Journal of Interprofessional Care*.

Ivan Koppel is senior partner in an inner-city general practice in London, whose work is based on close collaboration between different professional and occupational groups. He also holds a post of Principal Lecturer at the School of Integrated Health, University of Westminster, where he is involved in teaching on the range of interprofessional courses. His research interest is in analysis of discourses in continuing and interprofessional education.

Hugh Barr is Emeritus Professor of Interprofessional Education in the School of Integrated Health at the University of Westminster, Visiting Professor in Interprofessional Education in the School of Health and Social Care at the University of Greenwich, President of the UK Centre for the Advancement of Interprofessional

Education (CAIPE) and Editor-in-Chief of the *Journal of Interprofessional Education*. He was formerly an Assistant Director of the then Central Council for Education and Training in Social Work.

The Series

Promoting partnership for health

Health is everybody's responsibility: individuals, families, communities, professions, businesses, charities and public services. It is more than prevention and cure of disease. It is life-fulfilling for the well-being of all. Each party has its role, but effective health improvement calls for partnership, more precisely for many partnerships, which bring them together in innovative and imaginative ways. The scope for this series is correspondingly wide.

Successive books will explore partnership for health from policy, practice and educational perspectives. All three drive change. Policy presses the pace of reform everywhere, but change is also driven by the demands of practice, triggered by economic and social trends, technological advance and rising public expectations. Education responds, but also initiates, as a change agent in its own right.

Progressive health care is client centred. The series will wholeheartedly endorse that principle, but the client is also relative, citizen, client and consumer:

- Relative sustaining, and sustained by, family
- Citizen working for, and benefiting from, community, country and comity of nations
- Client of countless professions
- Consumer of health-enhancing or health-harming services

A recurrent theme will be the roles and responsibilities of professions, individually and collectively, to promote and sustain health. The focus will be on the health and social care professions, but taking into account the capability of every profession to improve or impair health. The responsibility of the professions in contemporary society will resonate throughout the series, starting from the premise that shared values of professionalism carry an inescapable obligation to further the health and well-being of all.

Each book will compare and contrast national perspectives, from developing and so-called developed nations, set within a global appreciation of opportunities and threats to health. Each will be driven, not simply by self-evident scope for one nation to learn from another, but also by the need to respond to challenges that pay no respect to national borders and can only be addressed by concerted action.

Partnership has become so fashionable that it is tempting to assume that all reasonable men and women will unite in common cause. Experience teaches otherwise: best laid plans too often founder for lack of attention to differences which can bedevil relationships between professions and between organisations. This series will not be starry-eyed. It will alert readers to the pitfalls and to ways to avoid them.

The three books introducing the series focus on collaborative working and learning between services and between professions in health and social care. In the first, Meads & Ashcroft (2005) find collaboration critical to effective implementation of health care reforms around the world. In the second, Barr *et al.* (2005) make the case for interprofessional education as a means to promote collaborative practice, corroborated by emerging evidence from systematic searches of the literature. In the third, this book, we marry evidence with experience, to assist teachers to develop, deliver and evaluate interprofessional education programmes. All three books transcend professional, organisational and national boundaries to share experience as widely as possible for the common good, as they set the tone for the series.

Hugh Barr
Series Editor
October 2004

List of other books in this series

Barr, H., Koppel, I., Reeves, S., Hammick, M. and Freeth, D. (2005) *Effective Interprofessional Education: Argument, Assumption and Evidence*. Blackwell Publishing, Oxford.
Meads, G. & Ashcroft, J. with Barr, H., Scott, R. & Wild, A. (2005) *The Case for Interprofessional Collaboration*. Blackwell Publishing, Oxford.

Foreword

The major challenge ahead for all who are interested in, and concerned with, carrying forward interprofessional education (IPE) for collaborative patient-centred practice is to develop, deliver, sustain and evaluate the entire process. The tasks faced in meeting this challenge include establishing a foundation based on scholarship and research in post-secondary education and practice settings that speaks to, and affirms, the experimental basis of IPE. This foundation can then inform policy makers in education, health and social care about appropriate courses of action that may be taken, based on evidence that has appropriate breadth and depth.

The challenge has an international reach as governments around the world grapple with the most effective health and social care delivery systems, with knowledge of the economic constraints on ensuring such delivery. Although this book draws largely from experience and expertise in the United Kingdom, its reach is clearly global.

IPE is **not** a synonym for teamwork, neither is it a synonym for collaborative practice. The breadth of IPE is slowly coming to be realized as a complex puzzle whose pieces intersect in many places and across many jurisdictions. Understanding IPE calls on not only the scope of health and social care professions, but also the academic basis of, for example, anthropology, sociology, geography, philosophy, economics, management and others. As the authors of this book show, interprofessionality is always about collegiality.

As an understanding of IPE develops, those who engage in its practice will be called upon to build tools to ensure that it is both successful and effective. The result of such efforts will be to ensure that IPE is absorbed into the body politic of disciplinary education as part of the natural education and training of all health and social care professionals.

At the centre of the concern of IPE must be the individual receiving care, followed by families and caregivers, and then the community in which care is provided. Each of these entities requires that we establish approaches that, as the authors say, 'realize the full potential of interprofessional education as a means for improving collaboration.'

How to approach IPE – a student, educator, administrator or policy maker requires information that is timely, easily accessible, informative and above all, practical. Illustrating 'how to' is a major challenge, since the facets of IPE needing to be demonstrated range from curricular development, through team preparation, to discussions of common language – and more, all of which are ultimately underpinned by the legal and ethical parameters of IPE.

The development of conditions for effecting IPE has depended largely on qualitative narratives from which object lessons have been drawn that focus attention on each of the components (and others mentioned above). Quantitative data has been slower to accumulate, partly because of the breadth of the scholarly base from which to articulate experimental methodologies. The psychology of organisational management has been of fundamental importance in informing change in team development, but, as has been shown in innumerable studies, the health care team is in many ways vastly more complicated than the team required, for example, to build a car. Although the application of team building theory has met with great success in manufacturing industries, it has proven difficult to implement in health care. Some of the reasons for this include, on the one hand, the false assumptions practitioners in specific professions hold about each other's knowledge and skills, and, on the other hand, the status and gender disparities that exist across professions. Historically, 'health' has been couched in biomedical terms. Little recognition has been given to the psychosocial aspects of health, and time after time the traditional roles of patient and provider have been reinforced. For clear reasons, those professions that have historically held dominant positions are reluctant to change. Yet, thankfully, over the past two decades health and social care practices have begun to change so that many of these difficulties are now being tempered thus making interprofessional collaboration not only a possibility but, in most health and social care settings, a distinct probability.

Given that the notion of 'teamwork' in health care is at least 100 years old, why should it have taken so long to become an established part of the parlance of health and social care? Better patient care ('evidence-based practice') is now seen as the desirable end towards which collaboration is aspiring, rather than the 'team' being seen as an end in itself. Such a view has not been reached without extensive discussions and debate about the meaning of 'interprofessional team' within health and social care settings. It is NOT always the case that health and social care teams are what they think they are, or operate as they think they should.

As anyone who has attempted to develop a team knows, simply getting its members to a common understanding of its goals and objectives is fraught with those occasions when intercultural variables have to be unpacked – an area of study that still deserves intensive examination.

One of the major stumbling blocks to effective collaboration, as most practitioners know, is poor communication. Frequently, in health and social care teams, this poor communication results from a lack of understanding of professional differences (and in many cases, of professional similarities). The difference between physician and nurse communication is often cited as an example of this lack of understanding of professional differences. We need to listen with a third ear in an effort to overcome miscommunication. Learning to reflect on and listen to the values and voices of one's professional colleagues makes excellent sense, but advice is not always heeded. And listening to the patient is only now becoming a central focus for health and social care professions. The education of health professionals has been remiss in its approach to teaching the skills necessary to communicate *between* professionals – it is to be hoped that educators will pay close attention to the suggestions provided in this book, and develop opportunities that carry this vision into not only classrooms, but also clinical contexts.

Learning effective collaboration requires more than sitting through a course and role-playing in a group. It requires both a personal transformation in view and a change in professional identity. To achieve the larger goal requires what might (erroneously) be seen as sacrifice. Building the larger cognitive and value maps require many things, not the least of which is a time in which to reflect on the changes taking place in self. Here the various metaphors used by the various professions in collaboration can serve as a powerful set of images to point out the inherent values of each viewpoint. Journaling and case discussions are the sorts of mechanisms that help achieve this desirable end.

Much has been written about leadership, in very many different contexts and it is clear that the health and social care setting is as needful of good leadership as elsewhere. To lead is to move forward – a point clearly made by the authors of this book, and one not to be belaboured here. How well a team handles conflict and the manner in which it solves problems are good indicators of either its functional or dysfunctional nature. It has to learn not only how to control conflict, but also about how to use it to promote interprofessional problem solving.

The challenges of pedagogy posed for the teaching and learning of interprofessional collaboration are more complex by far than those posed for teaching a course in English. The relationship between teaching and learning in a collaborative environment calls for all members to constantly be both teaching and learning – no easy matter. It is the experiential learning process that is fundamental to the teamwork process – learning by doing, by working with others. In grappling with issues that need resolution, the very difficult question of evaluation, taken in its broadest sense, needs clarification. How do we know that learning is occurring? If it is, what kind of learning is taking place? If it takes place, how do we measure its effectiveness – just following its occurrence? And what about 10 years hence? What metrics are best suited to evaluation of 'inter' methodologies? Because of the dynamic nature of teams, providing opportunities for lifelong learning is now a major goal for employers in the health care sector. What indeed is experiential learning?

This is a wonderfully useful 'workbook' for anyone contemplating (or even active in) IPE collaborative learning initiatives. The writing is clear, the book is replete with defining illustrative material, and there is a mass of solid, practical advice. Although interprofessional education has taken long strides in the past 15 years, it still has some way to go before it achieves the goals set by its scholars to date. This book assures that the strides will quicken, and the distance to the end goal of collaborative patient-centred practice will rapidly shorten.

John H.V. Gilbert, Ph.D.
Vancouver, B.C. Canada
February 2005

Acknowledgements

We draw extensively throughout this book on evaluations of interprofessional education conducted by fellow researchers at home and abroad, whose contribution we readily acknowledge. We have also valued support from our institutions – City, Westminster and, for much of the time, Oxford Brookes and Birmingham Universities.

Writing has been undertaken largely on the margins of busy workloads, encroaching on time to be with families, to whom we owe our thanks for their forbearance. A big thank you from Della to David, Rachael and Nadine, from Marilyn to James and Paul, from Scott to Ruth, William and Ewan and from Ivan to Vivienne and Gabriel.

Glossary

Action learning sets consist of series of facilitated meetings designed to allow the participants to explore real problems in an organisation. Members commit themselves to try out the identified solutions and report back.

Action research involves the researcher in working collaboratively with participants through cycles of *evaluation** and development to effect positive change in their relationships or practice.

Assessment is the process of judging the extent to which the participants have achieved the learning outcomes of a course. This process is also sometimes referred to as *evaluation*.

Cohort is the collective name for a group of students or research participants recruited to the course or study at one particular time.

Collaboration is an active and ongoing partnership, often between people from diverse backgrounds, who work together to solve problems or provide services.

Common learning is a concept that has a different meaning in different contexts. Originally, and still in its pure form, it refers to multi-professional education. However, common learning is also the name given to certain initiatives in *interprofessional education* in the UK.

Contact hypothesis suggests that friction between different social groups can be alleviated if they can interact with one another, provided certain conditions are met. These include equality of status, the need for members to work on common goals in a cooperative manner, and the need for members to focus on understanding differences and similarities between themselves.

Continuing professional development is learning undertaken after initial qualification for a particular job or profession, in order to maintain competence and develop capability.

Critical path analysis is a tool that assists with the scheduling and management of complex projects. It analyses the whole project into separate parts, scheduling them according to their estimated duration and establishing antecedent and postcedent relations between the different activities. The product is a network of

---

*Italicising indicates words in definitions in the glossary that are themselves in the glossary.

activities, which includes a critical path. Completion of the activities on the critical path are critical for successive phases of the project.

Curriculum is an overarching term for all those aspects of education that contribute to the experience of learning: aims, content, mode of delivery, assessment, and so on.

The **curriculum development team** (or development team) is responsible for developing a *curriculum*.

Enquiry-based learning (EBL) is an alternative term for *problem-based learning*, sometimes preferred to avoid negative connotations of the word 'problem'.

Evaluation is used to describe the processes of systematic gathering and interpretation of evidence, enabling judgement of effectiveness and value, and promoting improvement. Many evaluations have both *formative* and *summative* strands.

Discipline in this book means an academic discipline, such as psychology or biology, *and* subspecialties within professions, for example the disciplines of anaesthesia or radiology within the profession of medicine.

Formative evaluation of *interprofessional education* provides information and interpretations that can be used to make improvements *within* the development and delivery phases of an initiative.

Formal interprofessional education aims to promote collaboration and enhance the quality of care; therefore it is an educational or practice development initiative that brings people from different professions together to engage in activities that promote interprofessional learning. With formal *interprofessional education* the intention is for curriculum to achieve this aim (cf. *informal interprofessional education*).

Formative assessment of learning takes place during the educational initiative and its main purpose is to provide feedback to the learner of their progress.

Governance systems are those that enable an organisation to give an account of the way it manages itself. Clinical governance is a term used in the UK health service for systems that enable accountability of clinical services to assure their quality, safety and excellence.

Informal interprofessional education at its inception lacks the intention, and would fail to acknowledge, the interprofessionality and learning potential of the initiative. At any point in time after that it may be acknowledged that learning with, from and about each other is happening between participants. However, in many such initiatives, this remains unacknowledged or is only recognised on reflection: in and on the learning practice (cf. *formal interprofessional education*).

Integrated care pathways are locally agreed, patient-focused, *multi-professional* outlines of the anticipated care required for patients who share the same diagnosis or set of signs and symptoms. The pathway sets out the appropriate initiatives (based on clinical evidence and best practice) and the time frames in which these should be administered and the expected progress of the patient. The aim is to enhance coordination and consistency of care. They are also known as care maps, care profiles, care protocols, clinical paths, critical care pathways and multidisciplinary pathways of care.

Interprofessional education/training (IPE) describes, for the purpose of this book, those occasions when two or more professions learn with, from and about each other to improve collaboration and the quality of care. It is an initiative to secure *interprofessional learning* and promote gains through interprofessional collaboration in professional practice.

Interprofessional learning (IPL) is learning arising from interaction between members (or students) of two or more professions. This may be a product of *interprofessional education* or happen spontaneously in the workplace or in education settings (cf. *serendipitous interprofessional education*).

Interval data are a type of data in which the distances between numbers have meaning, for example the number of years a practitioner has been qualified.

Managed care developed in the USA to contain the runaway costs of medical care. A subscriber to a health plan will contract with a specific provider, such as a health maintenance organisation, within which the care and expenditure is monitored to avoid unnecessary investigation and treatment. Processes rely on the use of protocols and regular clinical and management reviews

Multi-professional education (MPE) is when members (or students) of two or more professions learn alongside one another: in other words, parallel rather than interactive learning.

Nominal data is a type of data in which numbers stand for names but have no order of value, for example: female $= 1$, male $= 2$.

Ordinal data is a type of data that ranks subjects in some kind of order, such as the scores on an attitude scale: very positive, positive, negative, very negative.

The **planning team** is responsible for the preparatory work that needs to be done before the development of an *interprofessional education* initiative. It is also called groundwork.

Practice placement is used as the generic term to cover clinical placement, attachment, rotation, fieldwork placement, practicum and other terms used by different professions to describe opportunities for students to apply and develop their learning in the workplace.

In **probability sampling** each 'unit' has a finite, known probability of being selected, enabling knowledge of how the sample is representative of the wider population. For example, with simple random sampling each unit has an equal probability of being selected; with cluster random sampling there is recognition of meaningful clusters within a population and random samples are taken within each cluster (see *sampling*, cf. *theoretical sampling*).

Problem-based learning (PBL) is a way of delivering a *curriculum* in order to develop problem-solving skills as well as assisting learners with the acquisition of necessary knowledge and skills. Students work cooperatively in groups to seek solutions to real world problems, set to engage students' curiosity and initiate learning of the subject matter.

Reflexivity is concerned with understanding the nature of the researcher and the relationship they hold with people they work with on an evaluation.

Sampling is the process of choosing a selection of 'units' or 'cases' (places, people, times, events, artefacts, etc.) from everything or everyone that might provide data and insights for an evaluation. Sampling is necessary for efficient use of resources. There are many forms of sampling, with two main paradigms: *probability sampling* and *theoretical sampling*.

Data **saturation** is reached in an enquiry using qualitative methods, when no new themes emerge from continuing cycles of data collection.

Serendipitous interprofessional education is unplanned learning between professional practitioners, or between students on *uni-professional* or *multi-professional* programmes, which improves interprofessional practice.

Staff development is the continued professional development of academic, practice and administrative staff through activities done by, and for them, to enhance their knowledge, skills and attitudes. Within universities it is often referred to as faculty development.

A **steering group** supports and advises complex, large and innovative projects, for example an undergraduate programme of *interprofessional* education for students from several different professions.

Summative assessment of learning takes place at the end of the educational initiative and its main purpose is to provide evidence, often for award purposes, of the changes in the knowledge and skills of the learner as a result of the initiative.

Summative evaluation judges the success of *interprofessional education* (ideally a multifaceted view with several outcome measures and attention to processes); thus accounting for resources and informing subsequent development and delivery.

A **syllabus** is a list of the topics covered during an education initiative and is often referred to as the course content. It is a subset of *curriculum*, not a synonym.

Teamwork is the process whereby a group of people, with a common goal, work together, often, but not necessarily, to increase the efficiency of the task in hand.

The logic of **theoretical sampling** contrasts with *probability sampling*, being less concerned with representativeness and focusing on the potential of a selected 'unit' to illuminate the evaluation questions or test an emerging analysis. Theoretical sampling might actively seek maximum variation and disconfirming cases; it could seek typical cases, unique cases, deviant cases, extreme cases or contrasting cases.

Triangulation is a technique for checking the integrity and sophistication of evaluation findings by examining data and interpretations from more than one vantage point. This may mean using more than one: evaluator, data collection method, data source, theoretical perspective, time point, or a combination of these. More trustworthy, comprehensive and complex insights should result.

Uni-professional education is members (or students) of a single profession learning together.

Validity is concerned with the accuracy of an evaluation. Different paradigms view validity differently because they have different conceptions of 'truth'.

This book is dedicated to the memory of John Hammick

Introduction

Effective interprofessional education for effective practice

Interprofessional education is being widely invoked as a means to improve practice in health and social care, which is demanding time, energy and resources in many countries. Interprofessional education must, however, be effective itself before it can further effective practice.

Interprofessional education is therefore critically important for most public, private and charitable services that have at their heart improving the well-being of individuals, families and communities. It is often the subject of national policy imperatives, to be enacted by service agencies and educational institutions, separately or together, but prompting issues that transcend national boundaries.

The effectiveness agenda is an established feature of the workplace, particularly, but not exclusively, in publicly funded services such as health and social care. This informs the interprofessional education agenda. The values that underpin assessment of performance, views on optimal approaches to getting the information on which judgements are made and the ways in which the results of an assessment are used can vary between professions or between organisations – effectiveness is a contested concept.

The effectiveness debate is here; many would say that it is here to stay. It behoves those of us interested in seeing it used (dare we say it) effectively to participate in the debate, on the one hand, about how interprofessional education can become more effective in furthering effective interprofessional practice and, on the other hand, how it can apply the same rigour in setting standards for effectiveness as that increasingly demanded of practice.

This book in the series

Our writing here, on developing, delivering and evaluating effective interprofessional education is intimately related to two other books in this series: Meads & Ashcroft (2005) and Barr *et al.* (2005). Each complements the others and paves the way for future contributions to the series. The aim, within all three texts, has been to establish a foundation for the forward thinking and practice of policy makers, programme planners, teachers and researchers. This book, along with its series' companions, is addressed to an international readership, recognising that interprofessional education permeates geographical and political boundaries.

We are mindful of international contributions to the body of knowledge about interprofessional collaboration and education and we have included several examples. However, we recognise that in our writing here, we have drawn most heavily from UK sources, reflecting the nature of our own experience and expertise, attained from, collectively, many years of diverse professional practice in UK higher education and health and social care. We brought to the task of writing this book backgrounds in cancer care, medical general practice and social work; experience of developing, delivering and evaluating interprofessional education; and perspectives from the disciplines of sociology, education and statistics. We have all been longstanding and active members of the UK Centre for the Advancement of Interprofessional Education (CAIPE). The value of the work of that organisation and the collegiality we have enjoyed with all its members have considerably added to our knowledge and shaped our thinking on interprofessionality.

We have all been fortunate to be involved with international colleagues and to learn from them the interprofessional developments taking place in their countries. We have also had the privilege of working alongside many UK colleagues as they develop, deliver and evaluate interprofessional education. You will read more about some of these throughout the book. We are grateful to have had this breadth of experience to draw upon and glad to have been able to include so many examples of robust curriculum development and delivery, and evaluation.

One of the companion books in this series, *The Case for Interprofessional Collaboration* by Meads & Ashcroft (2005) relates numerous examples worldwide. The other, *Effective Interprofessional Education: Argument, Assumption and Evidence* by Barr *et al.* (2005), compares the case made for such education with findings from our systematic review of evaluations of interprofessional education. Barr *et al.* (2005) and the present text have been written as single texts, all five of us contributing to their evolution and production. This collaboration is the natural extension of our joint enquiries, which began in 1997, to synthesise the evidence base for interprofessional education from published evaluations.

In the following chapters we aim to show you some ways of ensuring that interprofessional education is successful and effective: that is, well received and precipitating positive learning and change in respect of collaboration and teamwork. Our focus is on health and social care practitioners, but without excluding other professions or occupations that are relevant to care of patients, clients and communities. We offer practical help in establishing approaches that will realise the full potential of interprofessional education as the means of improving collaboration and, thus, creating better services for individuals, families and communities. This includes the key organisational and resource (financial and human) factors that underpin the successful delivery of effective education.

This book is an invitation to consider multiple viewpoints and multiple influences on interprofessional education, training and development (both personal and organisational). From this we anticipate that you will examine your own thinking on the topic. For brevity, from hereon the term education will be used to denote education, training and personal development.

A book to be used and consulted

It was our deliberate intention that the focus of the book should be on the discussion, elaboration and illustration of ways and means towards effective interprofessional education. This is a book to be used. It is a text for those working at arms-length from interprofessional education to dip into and reflect upon. For those with hands-on roles, it is a practice manual that should help you in two major aspects of your work. The planning, development and delivery of effective interprofessional education is the focus of Section II, while designing and implementing the evaluation of your work in a robust and pragmatic way is the focus of Section III. The practical help offered covers: selecting learning outcomes and substantive content for interprofessional education programmes, designing them to complement uni-professional and multi-professional education and building in systematic and relevant evaluation of their effectiveness.

As we wrote we had in mind two themes or master narratives:
The *practice* of developing, delivering and evaluating diverse curricula underpinned by the principles of interprofessional education.

Effectiveness and what this means in the development, delivery and evaluation of interprofessional education.

Alongside these consistent themes we worked to a set of objectives. These are set out in Box 1 and effectively summarise much of what we have said so far in this introduction.

Our readers

We anticipate that our readership will be diverse in respect of their experience, expertise, needs and role in the delivery of interprofessional education. You may be a teacher, trainer, manager, someone holding a request for funding for an interprofessional course, or a practitioner who has recognised a challenging issue

---

Box 1 Objectives of the book.

(1) To guide trainers and educators through the process of developing, delivering and evaluating interprofessional education for health and social care: whether as an entirely new development or by modification of existing provision.

(2) To draw attention to the current practice of interprofessional education, nationally and internationally, through examples and research-based models.

(3) To discuss the key organisational and resource (financial and human) factors underpinning the successful delivery of effective interprofessional education.

(4) To describe evaluation approaches and processes appropriate for different models of interprofessional education and provide guidance for the use of these in everyday practice.

within a practice setting that requires enhanced teamworking or inter-agency collaboration. You may be reading this book having had some years experience of working in higher education in your own profession and may have been involved in the development, delivery and evaluation of interprofessional educa-tion previously. You may now be involved with an entirely new development in interprofessional education or have been asked to support innovative continued professional development to enhance partnership working. Alternatively, it may be a modification of existing provision that is required. We anticipate that stu-dents studying the professional education of health or social care practitioners will also find aspects of our book useful.

Whatever your present role and interest in interprofessional education, if you are reading this then you are attracted and committed to enhancing the effective-ness of what you do or what you would like to do. The book's overall design allows you some choice about how you use it.

You may wish to start with the particular section or chapter that is most relevant to your present work. Having obtained what you want from a specific chapter we would encourage you to extend your reading into all the other important aspects we have written about.

Alternatively, perhaps in anticipation of your involvement with a programme of interprofessional education, you will find that reading the chapters in the order they are presented will deepen your knowledge and indicate the skills required for work you need to do. In addition, and in common with all manuals, we suggest that the book will serve as a reference source and aide-memoire as you and your colleagues plan, deliver and evaluate your interprofessional event or programme. So do please share this book with your colleagues. Consider using the ideas and case studies to stimulate discussion at team meetings. If you are planning workshops about interprofessional education you might like to build the group work around some of the key issues highlighted at the end of each chapter.

One question in your mind as you decide to devote more time and energy to exploring the book is probably why it is needed in the first place. You may be wondering if something like learning together to work together, that seems intuitively to make sense, cannot help but be effective. We expand on this import-ant issue later on. In particular, in Chapter two we set out our views on what effectiveness might mean in this context.

Our focus

We need to comment briefly on the type of interprofessional education that you will be reading about. Given that the book is about development, delivery and evaluation, it has only been possible to write about education that is overt, that is, planned in some way. We acknowledge that a great deal of interprofessional learning is implicit and informal. Spontaneous interprofessional learning makes an important contribution to professional development and to improving ser-vices. The hard work involved in this deserves to be valued and needs to con-tinue. However, such learning cannot be among the main foci of a book such as this. We must focus on tangible education that someone intends to develop, deliver and evaluate. Nevertheless, we recognise the importance of spontaneous interprofessional learning and so this has a place within the model of interprofessional education that we build in Chapter one.

In this book we will emphasise creating positive change through interprofessional education and avoiding negative outcomes. Our systematic review (see Barr *et al.*, 2005) failed to reveal any evaluations of interprofessional education that reported wholly negative outcomes. This was not unexpected given that papers with such findings are rarely offered for publication. However, there are studies that indicate mixed results or potentially negative outcomes. For example, interprofessional education can highlight previously covert problems within a care team; or the outcomes associated with interprofessional education can vary between cohorts of participants, or within the measures used to assess changes.

Papers that draw our attention to mixed or equivocal findings include Atwal (2002), whose study found that practitioners needed to think more about the collaborative efforts required to resolve differences of opinion and new problems that arose from an interprofessional initiative. Carpenter & Hewstone (1996) draw our attention to some worsening of attitudes among medical and social work students who attended two and a half days of shared learning. Singh (2002) reports major changes to team training to enhance family friendliness for mental health care practitioners, after findings showed that the initial interprofessional role-play training sessions had a negative impact on certain aspects of family friendliness. The changes made showed clear and sustained positive effects. See also Box 1.4 in Chapter one, van Staa *et al.* (2000). This book aims to help you to ensure your education plans are effective and that positive learning and change takes place.

A look inside

So, what awaits you in the three sections of the book? In Section I we discuss some fundamental aspects of interprofessional education and outline the meaning of effectiveness in the context of the social realism of achieving learning. Chapter one begins by looking at what it means to learn and work interprofessionally and then presents some models of education appropriate to this field of work. With these meanings and models in mind we then integrate the interprofessional and the educational elements. The result is an inclusive model of interprofessional education: one that accommodates diversity and difference, serves the present societal and political context well, and, importantly, is sufficiently flexible given the unknown nature of any future context.

In Chapter two we set out current perspectives on effectiveness, especially those models that are currently used in health and social care service and education settings. We argue for the importance of performance measurement approaches that are useful and practical, and that harmonise with, rather than intrude into, the working lives of staff. In this way our knowledge of what works, for whom, in what context, is likely to proceed at a pace to meet the demands for such evidence.

Chapters three to eight in Section II focus on developing and delivering interprofessional education. They are written for staff in education and health and social care services with responsibilities for these aspects of education. Interprofessional education may take many different forms and much of what you will read in Section II will be useful whatever the type of interprofessional education in which you are interested. Our aim has been to provide you with clear guidance on planning and developing an interprofessional curriculum. We set out ways to maximise the effort of the teams who design and document learning outcomes, course content, teaching and learning methods, the assessment strategy and so on.

In Chapter seven, we focus on staff development. Keeping in mind the diversity of the educators and trainers involved in interprofessional education, we discuss how to facilitate the development of the craft of teaching interprofessionally. The commentary includes the role of work-based learning, continuing professional development programmes and more formal award-based programmes for educators. We also take a look at ways to assist teaching staff in their journey across professional boundaries. Our position is that this is often painful and tortuous. It demands insight into personal and professional attitudes, language and values, sensitivity to deeply held beliefs in our colleagues, and a willingness to move forward differently.

Finally, in Chapter eight we turn to the nature of quality in interprofessional education, from two perspectives. One of these seeks to encourage reflection about the practice of developing and delivering interprofessional education. The other looks at the process of accreditation and approval by external agencies, including the regulatory bodies, across all types of interprofessional education. Importantly, we discuss the roles and responsibilities of those who offer advice to course development teams and/or control and participate in approval processes.

Section III concentrates on the evaluation of interprofessional education. We describe a range of evaluation approaches and discuss their appropriateness for different models of interprofessional education. The aim is to assist you in choosing tools with which you can work within the resources you have available for evaluation, and to provide guidance on using these and the information you collect in every day practice. As the book ends we look at the essential characteristics of sharing your evaluation work with others. Topics such as presenting and publishing research findings, reporting techniques in education evaluation and research, and writing for different audiences are covered.

Books provide linear and fairly tidy accounts of development and delivery, but the real world is complex and untidy. Strands in development and delivery overlap, recur and compete. Table 1 hints at this and shows how the chapters of this book form a whole, although it is still tidier than the real world. Those who develop, deliver and evaluate interprofessional education have to work creatively with complexity and conflicting demands.

Throughout the book we have selected examples that show innovation, typical cases, or highlight some of the key issues within the discourse of interprofessional

Table 1 Making it happen: developing, delivering and evaluating interprofessional education.

Development	Delivery	Further development and delivery
Understanding interprofessional education and adult learning (Chapters one and six) and thinking about effectiveness (Chapter two).	Process continues, understanding becomes more sophisticated, development team becomes more skilled.	
Planning team forms, this may simply be an interprofessional pair or, exceptionally, an individual champion (Chapter three). Undertakes groundwork: recognising presage, securing initial resources, outlining processes and curriculum possibilities (introduction to Section II and Chapter three). Pays attention to group processes, works with champions, forms interprofessional curriculum development team (Chapter four). Disbands with members, becoming champions, steering group members or members of the development team.	**Development team** pays attention to group processes and reviews the decisions and progress of the planning team (revisits Chapters one, two and three). Works with champions, advisors or reference groups (Chapter four). Agrees and communicates curriculum; secures resources; prepares or commissions learning materials (Chapters five and six). Delivers or commissions staff development and evaluation (Chapters seven, nine, ten and eleven). Seeks accreditation; pays attention to quality monitoring and improvement mechanisms (Chapters five and eight). Oversees pilot work (Chapters four, five and twelve).	**Development team** work continues, identifying and plugging gaps, addressing teething problems, taking time to stand back and review the bigger picture, daring to question the original assumptions and decisions, making necessary changes, continuing to communicate with champions, reference groups, staff, staff developers and evaluators.	**Development team** uses experience from delivery, knowledge from evaluation and knowledge of the wider context to make and evaluate incremental changes. It periodically reviews its group processes and membership.

Enthusiasm, expertise and influence of **champions** harnessed (Chapters four and ten)

Advice sought from current students, tutors, frontline service staff and service users (perhaps formed as reference groups) (Chapter seven)

Staff development (Chapter seven)

Evaluation and sharing the learning arising from development, delivery and evaluation (Chapters nine, ten, eleven, twelve and thirteen) education and its evaluation. They illustrate the diversity of such programmes across all sectors of health and social care, with learners from a wide range of professional backgrounds, of variable duration, with individual purposes and at all levels of education. Our selection is strongly linked to the societal and political drivers for increased collaborative practices which have been identified and discussed in the two companion books. In our presentation of the case studies we offer brief descriptions to set the scene and a critical friend commentary to draw out the key points of learning from each case. We anticipate that you will be able to identify aspects from several of the case studies that have features in common with the type of interprofessional education with which you are involved. All of this seeks to inform you, to guide you and to provide some degree of challenge to your thinking about interprofessional education. At the end of each chapter you will find key points and suggestions for further reading.

Section I
Interwoven Threads

Introduction

In the following two chapters we seek to establish a shared understanding with you, our reader, of the meaning of interprofessional education and its effectiveness. To do this we introduce a model that recognises the diversity and difference that characterise interprofessional education. Chapter one aims to give you a clearer idea about what interprofessional education is and how very different events and courses can legitimately be labelled interprofessional education.

In Chapter two we outline perspectives on effectiveness; especially those models currently used in education, health and social care. The context of measuring effectiveness in interprofessional education and the forces that act upon initiatives of this nature are explored. The aim is to provide you with some background knowledge of the present performance measurement agenda. We introduce some ways in which staff responsible for maximising the effectiveness of interprofessional education can work towards this important end point.

1 The Spectrum Illuminated

After defining interprofessional education, we build a model to illustrate the diversity of interprofessional education and training. The model is illustrated with embedded examples of meeting the learning and development needs of health and social care staff. It allows us to explain how we have delineated the types of interprofessional education that we focus on as we discuss their development, delivery and evaluation.

Interprofessional education: what is it?

Throughout this book we regard interprofessional education, training or development for health and social care as: 'Occasions when two or more professions learn with, from and about each other to improve collaboration and the quality of care'.[1]

Our view is that education and training are synonymous terms, meaning *planned initiatives*, designed to promote opportunities to learn and change. Personal development also happens through these learning opportunities. From hereon, we use education as the term for the ways and means by which learning is promoted. Unless we are quoting the work of others, we use the term interprofessional education.

Interprofessional education is an initiative to secure interprofessional learning and promote gains through interprofessional collaboration in professional practice. In the definition above, interprofessional education promotes *active* learning, *with, from and about others*. In our view, interprofessional learning does not occur when members of different professions simply listen to a presentation together, or *independently* access common learning materials. It arises from interprofessional interaction. It follows that the quality of that learning is influenced by the quality of the interaction. It also raises questions about why this very specific and resource-hungry type of education is so very important and why it is presently attracting so much attention.

---

[1] The words in this definition revert to those in an earlier version than the current definition used by CAIPE (1997). It reintroduces learning *with* each other to acknowledge the potential for generating new knowledge when issues are explored by two or more students learning together.

Interprofessional education: why promote it?

For over 30 years interprofessional education has been promoted in policy documents as a means to enhance collaboration, reduce service fragmentation and promote high quality client care (for example, DHSS, 1974; WHO, 1998; DoH, 2001; Health Canada, 2003). The cumulative effect of these policies has been to create an impetus for developing interprofessional education. This has emerged in a wide variety of settings and in many different forms, as will become apparent as you read the examples in this book. But why, you may be asking, engage in interprofessional education at all?

The case rests on the argument that interprofessional learning promotes collaborative professional practice and a more holistic view of clients' or patients' needs. Barr (2002; pp. 8–14) provided a useful history of 'motives and movements' within interprofessional education in the UK, citing many examples. Some of the motives and movements identified are shown in Box 1.1. Our companion volume, *Effective Interprofessional Education: Argument, Assumption and Evidence* (Barr et al., 2005), takes a more detailed look at the arguments for engaging with interprofessional education.

Collaborative client-centred practice has many facets. These include effective communication between individuals and agencies; appropriate division of workload and responsibility; and recognising the expertise of all concerned. Insightful planning and reviewing of care, minimising duplication, and minimising errors of both action and inaction are equally important. We would argue that high quality collaborative practice can increase professional satisfaction and the intrinsic motivation of team members' roles, aiding retention and reducing burnout.

There is encouraging evidence that interprofessional education can produce the positive changes we alluded to in the previous paragraph. This is demonstrated by the wide range of examples included in subsequent chapters and discussed

---

Box 1.1   Some motives and movements for interprofessional education.

- Improving working relations amongst health, social care and sometimes other professions; and collective movements promoting shared resources
- Formulating regulatory and academic frameworks, in order to improve care and professional status
- Modifying negative attitudes and perceptions
- Addressing failures in trust and communication
- Securing collaboration to implement policies
- Improving services and effecting change
- Coping with needs that exceed the capacity of any one profession
- Enhancing job satisfaction and easing stress
- Increasing workforce flexibility
- Countering reductionism and fragmentation
- Integrating specialist and holistic care

more thoroughly in our companion volume (Barr *et al.*, 2005). However, many successful interprofessional education initiatives remain largely localised and, often, vulnerable when short-term investment or key people depart (to which we will return in Chapters four and ten). We should recognise that locally focused, grass-roots driven interprofessional education is often well received. It secures positive short-term outcomes precisely because it grows from and meets the needs of those involved. Such interprofessional education recognises and builds from the learners' starting points, founded on important educational principles (see, for example, Knowles *et al.*, 1998). Positive long-term outcomes are often more challenging to achieve, with organisational change required to embed interprofessional education and its benefits.

Interprofessional education: when should it happen?

In Section II we will look at selecting a positive balance between interprofessional education and other education and also the optimum timing and location of interprofessional education. Meanwhile, we want to draw your attention to the debate, particularly in relation to timing, amongst those engaging with interprofessional education for health and social care. Some argue for an emphasis on embedding interprofessional education in pre-qualification programmes to diminish the effect of negative professional socialisation. Others posit that interprofessional education should be undertaken after qualification when professional identity is more formed and learning can be more easily located in clinical practice. Both these views carry merit, but each is unnecessarily limiting. It would be a mistake to assume that students beginning a pre-qualification programme for their chosen profession do not bring with them stereotypes of their profession and of others. Their views are formed in the everyday world of personal experience and engagement with print, broadcast and web-based media.

It is important not to regard interprofessional education as something a learner experiences, maybe gains credit for, and then moves on from. Interprofessional education is a means of promoting effectiveness throughout working lives, a thread running through practitioners' professional development, shaped by personal role, service contexts and policy imperatives.

Throughout the book we represent this thread with case studies of interprofessional education in pre- and post-qualification courses, universities and workplaces, emphasising diversity, with examples from different contexts. Each of these examples of interprofessional education makes a valid contribution to enhancing practitioner competence in collaborative working for a particular client group. Collectively they support the case for thinking broadly: not restricting opportunities for interprofessional education to any particular educational or service setting, academic level, or designated groups of practitioners.

To reprise our argument, interprofessional education is an initiative to secure interprofessional learning, and through this to promote interprofessional collaboration and enhance professional practice in public services. The aims of interprofessional education are to improve:

- The effectiveness of care
- Stakeholders' perceptions of care
- Working lives (on which we elaborate in Barr *et al.*, 2005)

What is far less simple is attempting to represent the breadth and complexity of when, how, where and for whom interprofessional learning to achieve these aims might take place. We suggest a model of interprofessional education that initially, and in its simplest form, conveys that breadth. In this way interprofessional education can be seen as a spectrum in which all events that fit the definition we gave at the beginning of this chapter have a place.

A spectrum of interprofessional education

In the next few pages we build up our model of interprofessional education, progressively sharing with you its diversity and complexity. The result embraces all types of interprofessional education and sets out the range of choices available to those who are planning such an initiative. As you will see later, the model also allows us to recognise interprofessional education that occupies an important place off the spectrum.

Our model focuses solely on interprofessional education, in other words, the learning with, from and about each other described at the beginning of the chapter. This is different and distinct from multi-professional education. We are adopting CAIPE's definition of multi-professional education as follows: occasions when two or more professions are learning side by side for whatever reason (CAIPE, 1997). In contrast to interprofessional education, multi-professional education does not require interprofessional interaction to be embedded in the teaching and learning activities. Participants may share learning resources in the same physical space, or electronically. They will hear or see the same things, but without the structured opportunity to learn with, from and about each other. Nevertheless, bringing members (or students) of different professions together for multi-professional education is quite likely to precipitate some interprofessional learning, however implicit and serendipitous. We will return to this shortly. First let us turn to Figure 1.1, the core of our model.

In Figure 1.1 the rectangle, with its progressive degree of visibility, symbolises planned education or training. It is a 'visible spectrum' of interprofessional education (just as a rainbow shows the range of colours within the visible spectrum of light). The diagram represents a continuum along which all planned interprofessional initiatives can be placed. The depth of shading represents the emphasis on interprofessional education. The diagram is most easily read from

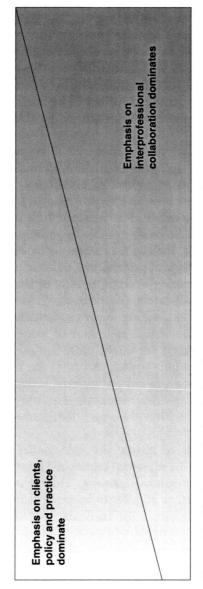

Figure 1.1 The interprofessional education spectrum.

right to left, remembering that everything within the rectangle is interprofessional education.

At the far right of the spectrum all the course or workshop content is explicitly interprofessional. People are brought together to learn with, from and about each other and about interprofessional collaboration as a means of improving care. There will need to be one or more vehicle for this learning, for example case studies, problem-based learning or shared practice learning. Moving towards the left, the dominance of the focus on interprofessional collaboration recedes. It is still intended that participants will learn with, from and about each other, improving their subsequent collaboration and care, but other learning outcomes are increasingly important. The dominant focus will be on, for example, developing technical knowledge or practical skills to address particular conditions such as diabetes or child neglect.

At the extreme left of the interprofessional education spectrum the content may be relevant to learners from a number of professions or disciplines[2]. Interprofessional learning may not be made explicit in, for example, the advertising of the event or course materials. However, an interprofessional focus, as a small part of a multifaceted agenda, will still reside in the heads of those planning and delivering the educational programme, becoming visible to participants as the programme unfolds. Interactive elements, such as brainstorming or small group discussions, will naturally draw on the range of professional and disciplinary expertise within the learner group, thus promoting a certain amount of interprofessional learning.

Pure multi-professional education (learning alongside one another, without planned interaction, aimed at securing improved collaborative practice) would therefore lie just outside the visible spectrum of interprofessional education, as Figure 1.2 shows. Arguably, we might place uni-professional education in multi-professional settings a little further out from the IPE spectrum rectangle; then uni-professional education in uni-professional settings still further out. For simplicity on the diagram multi-professional and uni-professional education have been placed together within the space that surrounds the spectrum of interprofessional education.

The two encircling bands of mostly invisible matter surrounding planned educational events in Figure 1.2 represent unplanned interprofessional education: first, serendipitous interprofessional learning. This is the unplanned learning with, from and about each other in order to improve collaborative care that may occur at any time when members (or students) of two or more professions interact. This interaction may take place in the workplace, in educational settings, or in social spaces. This is learning in the midst of the action of providing care and delivering a service. It is also the implicit learning running parallel with planned education; perhaps during coffee breaks or learner-instigated diversions during small group activities. It is a by-product of multi-professional education.

---

[2] In this book we shall use discipline to mean academic discipline, such as psychology or biology, *and* subspecialties within professions, for example the disciplines of anaesthesia or radiology within the profession of medicine.

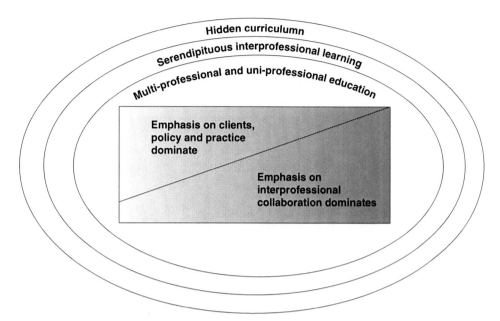

Figure 1.2 Detail of the interprofessional education spectrum in its wider context.

At this point you could stop and think about what types of serendipitous interprofessional education occur within your spheres of practice. Do you want them all to remain serendipitous, implicit and nearly invisible? Would there be advantages in trying to move some of this activity to the visible spectrum of planned interprofessional education? What would be the costs of doing this?

We are not arguing that serendipitous or implicit interprofessional education should be discouraged. Whenever it occurs, wherever it happens and whoever is involved there is no doubt that it makes a contribution to what practitioners know about working interprofessionally and fully deserves recognition.

The other invisible matter noted in Figure 1.2 is the hidden curriculum: un-planned learning that is not immediately recognised as such. We will return to the hidden curriculum in the introduction to Section II. Meanwhile, Figure 1.3 further illustrates the visible spectrum with a series of examples. On the left of the spectrum, overall profession-specific learning outcomes are dominant, interpro-fessional learning outcomes are only a minor part of a much longer course. For example, award-bearing programmes may include interprofessional education modules such as the one for pre-qualification social work students and mental health nursing students that is described in Box 1.2.

Further along the spectrum, some interprofessional education is explicitly designed to pay equal attention to, on the one hand, expertise for a particular area of professional practice and on the other hand, interprofessional collabor-ation. The M.Sc. in Society, Violence and Practice (Box 1.3) developed at City University, London, to promote expert practice in caring for survivors of violence of all types is a good post-qualification example of this. Near the extreme right of

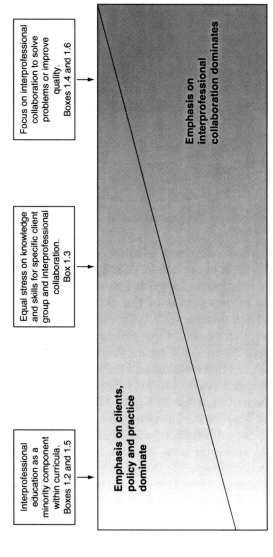

Figure 1.3 Key examples on the interprofessional education spectrum.

> **Box 1.2** Interprofessional education as a minority component within uni-professional curricula: collaborative practice in mental health, University of York, UK. (Departments of Health Science and Social Policy and Social Work, University of York.)
>
> This module for social workers and mental health nurses studying for their initial professional awards has been developed through a two-year project co-managed by departments of health sciences and social policy and social work. Funded by the Higher Education Funding Council for England Fund for the Development of Teaching and Learning, it brings these students together for the first time.
>
> The module aim: to develop knowledge, attitude and skills required for interprofessional working in a needs-led service, is based on the premise that mental health services are undergoing unprecedented organisational change and are complex and diverse. This demands good teamworking, coordination and information exchange. There is evidence that these crucial features of an effective mental health service have been absent in a number of failures of community care.
>
> The module is compulsory for third-year students on the Diploma in Nursing Studies (mental health branch) and optional for second-year students on the Master's in Social Work.

the interprofessional education spectrum, bringing people together to improve their teamworking and collaborative practice dominates the planned learning outcomes. Box 1.4 describes this type of interprofessional education developed for the staff of a palliative care unit in the Netherlands.

As the preceding examples have begun to show, the planned learning experiences within our spectrum of interprofessional education occur at different levels

> **Box 1.3** M.Sc. in Society, Violence and Practice, City University, London, UK.
>
> This part-time modular programme focuses on the delivery of expert practice in caring for survivors of violence (e.g. rape, child abuse, domestic and road traffic violence). It is a product of collaboration between health professions, the police service and the voluntary sector. Its development benefited from the engagement of people with current frontline experience of caring for survivors of violence and their loved ones, as well as people whose daily frontline experience had to some extent been supplanted by developing expertise in educational or senior managerial roles. Enquiry-based learning, supplemented by other forms of interactive learning, provides a good balance of structure and flexibility for the experienced practitioners who join this programme. Two of the programme modules have also been offered at B.Sc. level.

(Continues)

Sully (2002) provided a reflective account of the macro and micro group processes that evolved during the establishment of this programme, drawing attention to psychological safety and effective working practices for this partnership development, particularly a shared and upheld task focus; also the role of key champions and networks, including international collaboration. She stressed the importance of building upon prior course development, while retaining the courage to introduce new practices where necessary.

Sully identified the maintenance of boundaries and the clarification of language as major challenges, requiring skilful group facilitation. She noted that many of the facets of successfully developing and delivering this interprofessional programme mirrored the processes and skills required to deliver appropriate interdisciplinary services engaged in collaborative working with survivors of violence.

This example of interprofessional education is particularly important to us in representing the mid point of our spectrum: the knowledge skills and attitudes required for expert practice in this field and the interprofessional nature of the programme are equally important. This is because high quality interprofessional practice is vital in expert practice with survivors of violence. However, this trail-blazing course remains the exception rather than the norm in continuing professional development for practitioners working with this client group.

and in many different settings. They include courses leading to first or second degrees and/or professional registration; modules within learning programmes; short continuing professional development courses, including individual workshops; action-learning sets; and so on. Interprofessional learning occurs in

Box 1.4 An interprofessional workshop in palliative care, the Netherlands.

van Staa and colleagues (van Staa *et al.*, 2000) report on an interprofessional programme for 24 staff working in a palliative care unit in the Netherlands. Unit staff from dietetics, medicine, nursing and physiotherapy initially participated in a three-day residential course that aimed to enhance their collaborative work through a series of teambuilding sessions. The workshop was followed up by weekly team support meetings to help consolidate their interprofessional learning experiences. A longitudinal evaluation of the effects of this programme, including questionnaires, interviews and documentary data, revealed that staff reactions were mixed. While they enjoyed and valued this interprofessional learning and felt that the programme had created a more open atmosphere between staff members, it was also noted that members still encountered problems in their collaborative work, especially around a lack of clearly defined roles. The authors suggested that further team-based education would be required to overcome the persistent problems around role clarity between unit staff.

classrooms and within practice settings. Box 1.5 gives details of a practice-based example for pre-registration students and Box 1.6 shows an interprofessional approach to continuous quality improvement in the workplace.

Further examples, demonstrating the variety of interprofessional education, will be found throughout the book. The subject matter, planned learning outcomes and teaching and learning strategies all play a role in identifying where a particular education programme is located on the spectrum. As you will read later these are fundamental elements of the overall package of education, for which the overarching term *curriculum* is widely used. We will return to curriculum at the beginning of Section II.

Box 1.5   Training the dental team together in outreach placements: University of Sheffield, UK (The Team Training Programme Management Group, School of Clinical Dentistry, University of Sheffield and Barnsley, Rotherham & Doncaster Community Dental Services (CDS), Bury CDS, Hull Dental Access Centre, Lincoln Dental Access Centre, Liverpool CDS, North Yorks CDS (Northallerton), North Derbyshire CDS (Chesterfield), Rochdale & Bury CDS, Sheffield CDS, Tameside CDS (Ashton)).

Outreach practice-based interprofessional education plays a role in the pre-registration studies of dental health care students at Sheffield University. The initiative arose from recognition that dental teams need to develop and expand to meet the needs of all communities: challenges that are at the heart of UK Government policy (Department of Health, 2002). The aim is to develop and embed an interprofessional approach to dental education through placements for teams of dental undergraduates, hygienists, therapists and nurses in NHS primary care.

The success of a spring 2003 pilot of the initiative (20 undergraduate and therapy students in a six-week block placement in primary care clinics, in areas of need, supervised by local dentists), was followed by a half-cohort study in 2004. These were used to inform further developments for full implementation.

The 2003 pilot study explored students' experience through semi-structured interviews. (Interviewers were independent of the course team.) Triangulation included scrutiny by a second observer, a questionnaire survey and peer-run focus groups. Overall, students were very positive about the potential role of outreach training in dental education and the benefits of working as part of a team. They suggested common theory sessions to promote mutual understanding and better team working once qualified.

A team training group drives the initiative, developing training packages for supervising dentists, encouraging the production of learning materials for placement students and coordinating the changes needed to ensure coherence with other parts of students' programmes.

Box 1.6   An interprofessional course for continuous quality improvement
in general practice, UK.

Cox *et al.* (1999) provide an example of how interprofessional education
underpinned the development and delivery of a continuous quality improvement initiative for general practitioners and receptionists working in the UK.
Difficulties related to an increasingly high workload for the receptionists at
one practice, combined with regular difficulties obtaining repeat prescriptions
from general practitioners. This resulted in patient complaints about delays in
receiving their prescriptions. Working with a continuous quality improvement facilitator, the senior general practitioner, the practice manager and
three receptionists began to resolve this problem through the use of a plan-
do-study-act approach. During a series of interprofessional meetings, the
group established a more systematic approach to their repeat prescription
system, where information was stored electronically and where general practitioners could be contacted at specific times for authorising repeat prescriptions. Following its implementation, it was found that the prescription system
became more efficient. Indeed, it was found that 99% of prescriptions were
ready within 48 hours and that patient complaints were significantly reduced.
The authors conclude that an interprofessional approach to continuous quality
improvement can be particularly effective in allowing staff to share approaches to their work and generate ideas for change and improvements in
their practice.

Our selection of examples for the spectrum model was made in relation to the
concept of intentionality. The education in the examples we describe is visible,
the learning was intended and planned and, some, if not all of it, was designed to
be interprofessional. This does not guarantee that positive interprofessional learning will occur. It does presume that the means to promote interprofessional
learning will have been planned, with careful choice of relevant topics, suitable
learning resources and appropriate teaching methods.

The types of interprofessional education that have a place between the points
defined by our selected case studies are enormously varied. While many
examples of interprofessional education will be discrete events or courses this
may not always be the case. Towards the left of the spectrum the interprofessional
learning intention is often secondary to other aspects of the education event. In
such cases it may be difficult to assess the significance of this secondary intention
during the early stages of the development. We would encourage workshop
facilitators and training event managers to think much more about the interprofessional element during the planning stage, since this has the potential to enhance interprofessional learning.

The types of interprofessional education we selected to illustrate our model are
examples; the list is not exhaustive. There are slightly different versions of each
type, all making a valuable contribution to improving collaborative working

across many health and social care services worldwide. They all, however, have two common features. They are based on the values and principles that underpin achieving interprofessional learning *and* they use a curriculum to communicate their way towards this end: we will work more at this in Section II.

In conclusion: the uniqueness of interprofessional education

Having demonstrated huge variety within learning initiatives that can be termed interprofessional education, it is useful to consider what is unique about interprofessional education. In part this brings us back to the definition of interprofessional education that opened the chapter. We believe that the intention to learn with, from and about members of a different professional tribe is a defining and unique feature of interprofessional education. From this, it follows that achievement of interprofessional learning involves understanding a different professional culture and its associated customs, practices and language.

The heterogeneity (diversity) of learner groups brings practical challenges for teachers and facilitators. The learners will start with different sets of prior knowledge, different expectations about the ways in which education should be conducted, and, very probably, different aspirations about the benefit that might arise from engaging with interprofessional education. Of course, heterogeneous learning groups also offer unique teaching and learning opportunities that can be used creatively by planners and participants. These challenges and opportunities of heterogeneity extend beyond the composition of learner groups, to teachers, planners, budget holders and regulators. They provide a need and focus for staff development. We will focus on staff development in Chapter seven.

Key points

- Positive learning and change are the *raison d'être* of educational initiatives.
- Effective interprofessional education will maximise positive and minimise negative learning.
- Interprofessional education is an initiative to secure interprofessional learning and through this to promote interprofessional collaboration and enhance professional practice in public services.
- The aims of interprofessional education are to improve:

    - the effectiveness of care
    - stakeholders' perceptions of care
    - working lives

- Interprofessional education is conceptually distinct from multi-professional education and uni-professional education, although often combined with them.

- The quality of the interprofessional interaction is a major contributor to the quality of the interprofessional learning.
- Interprofessional education is not a one-off initiative: it is a means of promoting good care and professional satisfaction throughout working lives.

2 Effectiveness

We start from the assumption that anyone developing or delivering interprofessional education would wish it to be effective. We argue that this warrants explicit attention to the nature of effectiveness and those conditions that may promote effective interprofessional learning.

What is effective?

An initiative may be considered to be effective if it:

- Has (on balance) positive outcomes
- Has an acceptable cost
- Is without unacceptable side effects

For interprofessional education positive outcomes might include: positive reactions to the learning experience; new knowledge and skills for teamwork and wider collaboration; improved attitudes towards collaboration or colleagues' contributions to care. In addition, there might be more or better collaborative behaviour, or changes in the organisation or delivery of care that benefit patients and clients, families and communities. Our development of the Kirkpatrick[1] typology of outcomes (Barr *et al.*, 2000) acknowledged this breadth. We return to the importance of considering all of the outcomes in a number of places in this book.

Costs may be financial, and we consider cost effectiveness as part of the wide effectiveness discourse below. Alternatively, they may take the form of time, space and other physical resources. There may also be a loss of status. Coping with, and working to resolve, challenge and change inevitably brings emotional costs. Stressful interpersonal relations within the workplace can result from the assimilation of ideas from interprofessional education by an enthusiastic convert and subsequent blocking of their desires to establish collaborative practice by unconvinced colleagues. Unacceptable side effects of unsuccessful interprofessional education could include the development or hardening of negative stereotypes and antipathy towards further interprofessional learning.

---

[1] Kirkpatrick's 1967 model is discussed at length in Thackwray (1997).

Faulty or dangerously incomplete learning may also be transferred to professional practice: an unacceptable side effect of any educational initiative, not only inter-professional education. We will return to costs and benefits in the following chapters.

It is sensible and fair to assume that anyone developing or delivering inter-professional education would wish it to be effective. We argue that this warrants explicit attention to the nature of effectiveness and to those conditions that may promote effective interprofessional learning. Effectiveness is a slippery concept. It is possible to interpret it in a variety of ways. The following sections first consider the broader context of multiple discourses of effectiveness. We then go on to discuss effectiveness within interprofessional education.

Wider discourses of effectiveness

Any consideration of effectiveness in interprofessional education needs to recog-nise the presence and influence of mechanisms to assess effectiveness in educa-tion and in health and social care. Interprofessional education provided by universities and colleges is subject to approval within multi-professional or uni-professional programmes as we discuss in Chapter eight. Approval of these programmes must take into account findings from clinical governance and the evidence-based practice context in which students may be employed. Interprofes-sional education must, in addition, take into account collaborative practice and strategies for modernisation expected in those services.

Agendas invoking modernisation often assume the readiness of professions to pull together, discounting any potential tensions and their adverse effects. Inter-professional education can be instrumental in effecting change, for example through total quality management and continuing quality improvement initia-tives as Box 1.6 demonstrates. It can also be remedial if and when tension is generated. This is a persuasive argument (but not, of course, the only one) for continuing with interprofessional education initiatives in anticipation of inescap-able tensions in working life and the need for it to be at the ready.

Education in practice is an absolutely essential part of all programmes for health and social care practitioners and there is a resurgence of the expectation that teaching will be delivered by jointly appointed service and education staff. The development, delivery and, therefore, the approval, of effective interprofes-sional education is almost always, some would say *should* always be, a partner-ship between service and education institutions and colleagues.

Interprofessional education responds to findings from reviews of service effect-iveness and prepares its students to engage in such reviews. We have therefore included summaries of five of the more common review processes connecting each to interprofessional education. Each has individual features. Most share some common characteristics. The choice of what measures of effectiveness to use is often dependent upon professional and political contexts. All five are mechanisms to assess whether initiatives in care sector services, including the learning opportunities they offer, achieve effectiveness, namely:

(1)   Clinical effectiveness
(2)   Evidence-based practice
(3)   Cost effectiveness
(4)   Professionalism and ethical practice
(5)   Clinical governance

If we had more space in this chapter we would include other equally appropriate examples, such as audit, appraisal and revalidation. A lack of space also prevents any discussion of the role and value of comparative effectiveness.

Another vital element in the effectiveness agenda is the difference in approach that is needed when assessing short- or long-term effectiveness. We return to this later in this chapter in a discussion of a typology of outcomes to measure the effectiveness of interprofessional education for health and social care practitioners, and again in Section III. But first we will take a brief look at our five examples of assessing effectiveness.

(1) Clinical effectiveness

In the UK, clinical effectiveness became an important feature of health care policy from the mid-1990s onwards. Landmark documents included *Improving Clinical Effectiveness* (NHSE, 1993) and *Promoting Clinical Effectiveness* (NHSE, 1996). The latter defined clinical effectiveness as:

> 'The extent to which specific clinical initiatives, when deployed in the field for a particular patient or population, do what they are intended to do – i.e. maintain and improve health and secure the greatest possible health gain from available resources.' (NHSE, 1996)

In this model effectiveness is more down to earth than efficacy. Efficacy is the power or potential to produce a desired effect, often determined under experimental conditions. Effectiveness is about what is actually achieved within the complexity of the real world, which more and more often demands that practitioners collaborate and in which students gain interprofessional learning experience. Clinical effectiveness is also a process for continuous quality improvement rather than an intermittent measurement of achievement. Achieving effectiveness in the context of complexity and viewing improvement as a continuing process are also applicable to the field of interprofessional education.

Through its endeavour to take the service context into account, clinical effectiveness is inextricably linked to *evidence-based practice*.

(2) Evidence-based practice

Evidence-based practice seeks to bridge the gap between knowledge (usually derived from primary research or systematic reviews) and the consistent, rational application of that knowledge in daily practices of social care, health care, policy formation and education. The dominant discourse is evidence-based medicine (EBM), defined by Sackett *et al.* (1997, p. 71) as:

> 'the conscientious, explicit and judicious use of current best evidence in making decisions about the care of individual patients, based on skills which allow the doctor to evaluate both personal experience and external evidence in a systematic and objective manner.'

The importance of 'explicit and judicious use of current best evidence' is that it permits the considered use of many types of evidence when decisions are made about care. It also encourages scrutiny of the available evidence, naturally identifying gaps or other deficiencies and encouraging continuous quality improvement for services and continuing professional development for individuals. A number of settings, for example education, have developed the concept of using evidence as one of the tools that shape the way policy is made and implemented. This approach is described as evidence-informed policy and practice and has many similarities to the evidence-based movement. The Best Evidence Medical Education Collaboration, the Campbell Collaboration and the Evidence for Policy and Practice Information and Coordinating Centre all provide support for staff working to develop the evidence base in education and the social sciences (see website addresses at the end of this chapter). One key difference between such groups lies in the methods used to establish evidence and to judge its authority.

The contestable nature of evidence for practice impacts on interprofessional education in two main ways. First, the dynamics of interprofessional learning will be affected by participants' views of the nature of professional practice and its evidence base. Facilitators who anticipate this tension can plan to manage it creatively rather than allow it to become destructive. We will return to the importance of high quality facilitation in interprofessional education in Section II. Second, the contestable nature of evidence for practice impacts directly on the evaluation of interprofessional education. How you characterise effectiveness directly influences how you set about measuring it and whether you think you have found it. Evaluations of interprofessional education must always meet the needs of more than one profession. In fact it is often necessary to try to satisfy a wide range of stakeholders. We say more about this challenge in Section III.

(3) Cost effectiveness

Cost effectiveness or 'value for money' is a further strand in the discourse of effectiveness. It can be thought of as the ratio:

$$\frac{\text{Cost of a particular activity or initiative}}{\text{Value of outcomes attributed to the activity or initiative}}$$

The smaller this ratio, the better value for money is being obtained. In other words, the cost of the initiative will be as low as possible in relation to the value attached to outcomes. Cost–benefit ratios can vary greatly. They are very dependent on the definition and boundaries of the costs and benefits used in the calculation. This is very noticeable in the case of interprofessional education.

The direct monetary costs of interprofessional education fall on the purchasers of professional education. In the case of a block grant or a devolved budget it is the providers of professional education who must decide the appropriate proportion of fixed resources to allocate to interprofessional education. Other resource costs of interprofessional education fall on participating organisations and individuals. But where do the benefits of interprofessional education fall? The goal is that most benefits of interprofessional education fall in service delivery settings. With pre-qualification interprofessional education, in particular, it is easy to end up with virtually all costs in one accounting system and most benefits spread across a variety of balance sheets. Its paybacks are long-term and set in contexts that may be far removed from its point of delivery. While this temporal separation of costs and benefits applies equally to uni-professional education, established ways of doing things tend to be subject to less critical scrutiny than innovations.

(4) Professionalism and ethical practice

Effectiveness is entwined with the discourses of professionalism and ethical practice. Offering effective initiatives and treatments is an integral part of practitioners' duty of care towards patients and clients. Arguably, a commitment to professionalism and ethical practice demands ongoing attention to whether the initiatives you offer are effective and suited to their context. In the case of commissioning or providing interprofessional education, professionalism and ethical practice might be viewed as making robust defensible decisions, securing adequate resources and managing these wisely. Supporting participants and maximising the acceptability of the educational initiative among the relevant stakeholder are also duties of care. It is also important to evaluate processes and outcomes so that development can be encouraged and good practice can be shared.

(5) Clinical governance

Clinical governance was introduced as a statutory duty for UK National Health Service providers following the White Paper *A First Class Service* (Department of Health, 1998). Clinical governance is an umbrella term for a set of structures and processes that seek to guarantee high quality care, dependably delivered at a local level with equitable access, and to promote continuous quality improvement. To a great extent the concept of clinical governance drew together different perspectives on quality and effectiveness. Namely, local and national programmes of clinical audit; the development of National Service Frameworks for specific areas of care, which frequently emphasise the need for increased collaboration, and linking best evidence for clinical and cost effectiveness with services users' perspectives on service delivery. It also focused an increase in the attention given to risk management; and to implementing guidance from the National Institute for Clinical Excellence[2] (www.nice.org.uk); as well as supporting practice and professional development, including lifelong learning; valuing input from service users, health care professionals, support staff, managers, researchers, professional bodies, and NHS quality organisations such as the National Patient Safety Agency (NPSA). Clinical governance links the judgements and actions of individual health care practitioners with national standards and public accountability. Swage (2000, pp. 5–6) summarised four key issues in relation to this:

- Clear lines of responsibility for the quality of clinical care
- A comprehensive programme of quality improvement activities
- Clear policies aimed at managing risk
- Procedures for all professional groups to identify and remedy poor performance

The idea is to create an environment in which the collaborative pursuit of high quality care can flourish. To do this, as Degeling and colleagues (2004) remind, it is imperative that clinical governance includes not only risk management and quality matters, but extends into the work of all clinical professionals as teams. This makes clinical governance a natural focus for interprofessional education (see, for example, Box 2.1).

Box 2.1   Clinical governance and interprofessional education.

Reeves *et al.* (2000) describe a series of three interprofessional sessions for pre-registration house officers (junior doctors) and newly qualified nurses working in a London hospital, which were developed in response to the implementation of the UK's clinical governance policy (Department of Health, 1998). This policy stresses the need for evidence-based practice, increased clinical performance and teamwork. The sessions had three aims: to provide opportunities to address patient care issues in an interprofessional manner; to provide an educational programme that promoted an understanding of one another's professional roles; to promote better teamwork to improve patient care.

Each session lasted for two hours and focused on a separate issue: discharge planning, pain management and intravenous drug administration – areas in which local clinical audit data indicated the service could be enhanced. Participants undertook joint problem-solving activities based around a number of case scenarios and hands-on activities linked to setting up intravenous pumps. Clinical experts from a number of professions shared their perspectives during the group work and during the plenary feedback activity at the end of each session.

Findings from an evaluation of the programme revealed that participants enjoyed the sessions and felt their clinical and collaborative knowledge and skills had been enhanced.

---

[2] The social care equivalent of NICE is the Social Care Institute for Excellence (www.scie.org.uk).

The downside of effectiveness procedures and debates

If a continual quest to provide effective care or effective education is simply a facet of professionalism, arguably there would be no downside to effectiveness, but practitioners sometimes experience effectiveness procedures and debates as unsatisfying or even burdensome. For example, there are complaints that the dominant models of striving for effectiveness accentuate that which is easily measurable. Many aspects of care or education are difficult to measure directly and there are fears that these can be inappropriately downgraded.

Developing proxy measures and innovative ways of measuring can help, but portraying complexities and subtleties remains problematic. Strongly linked to this is the ability to communicate the messages from effectiveness measures in straightforward ways. Preference may be given to the impact of a pie chart, rather than allowing space for a narrative account which gives breadth and depth to the aspect of practice under scrutiny.

Of course, both learning and quality improvement should be continual processes for individuals and organisations, but people become jaded if processes are too burdensome, repetitive, or apparently yield little benefit. The processes and procedures advocated for the implementation of effectiveness may, over the long term, feel something like a treadmill of appraising, evaluating and measuring. Figure 2.1, taken from a UK example addressed to nurses, midwives and health visitors, shows the pathway towards clinical effectiveness and how many of its steps require staff to identify and appraise new knowledge. This learning activity may take precious time in the lives of busy staff. This does not make clinical effectiveness a bad idea, but it does highlight a need for attention to ways of maintaining commitment. These might include introducing opportunities for creativity in the processes, building from practitioners' natural interests and concerns, and prioritising strategically, because there will always be too much to be done.

Having established that effectiveness is a multifaceted and contestable concept, let us now return to effectiveness in the context of interprofessional education.

Effectiveness in interprofessional education

To reprise the argument that opened the chapter, effective interprofessional education will deliver positive outcomes, at acceptable cost, without unacceptable side effects. Questions that arise from this include: what is the nature of positive outcomes that might be delivered by interprofessional education, who should assess effectiveness and how it will be judged? Figure 2.2 explores the *who* and some questions they might ask. There may be additional stakeholders in your context. The questions they might ask will be related to that particular context. This is one area you, possibly with your colleagues, could spend some time considering at an early stage in the development of your course and its evaluation.

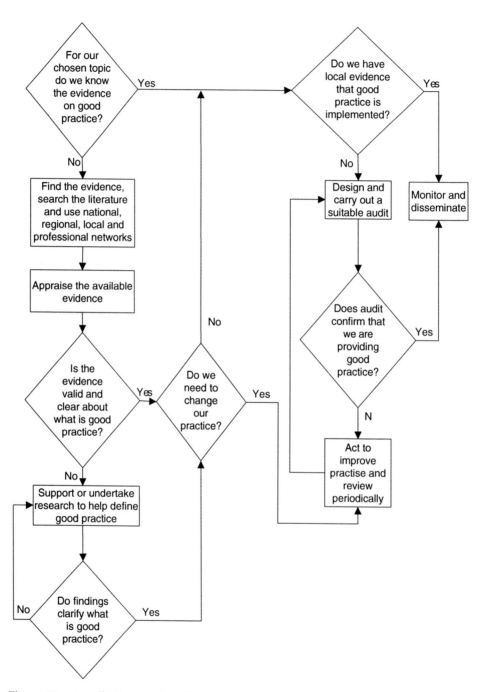

Figure 2.1 An effectiveness flowchart.

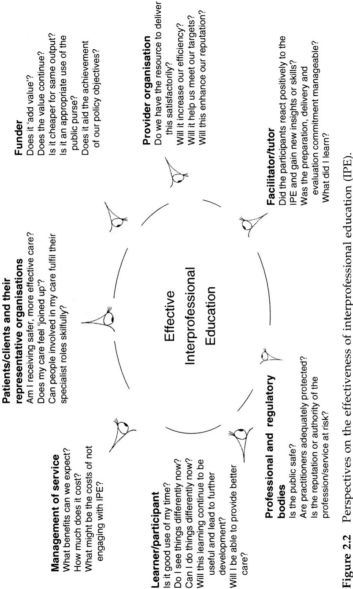

Management of service
What benefits can we expect?
How much does it cost?
What might be the costs of not
engaging with IPE?

Learner/participant
Is it good use of my time?
Do I see things differently now?
Can I do things differently now?
Will this learning continue to be
useful and lead to further
development?
Will I be able to provide better
care?

**Professional and regulatory
bodies**
Is the public safe?
Are practitioners adequately protected?
Is the reputation or authority of the
profession/service at risk?

**Patients/clients and their
representative organisations**
Am I receiving safer, more effective care?
Does my care feel 'joined up'?
Can people involved in my care fulfil their
specialist roles skilfully?

Effective
Interprofessional
Education

Funder
Does it 'add value'?
Does the value continue?
Is it cheaper for same output?
Is it an appropriate use of the
public purse?
Does it aid the achievement
of our policy objectives?

Provider organisation
Do we have the resource to deliver
this satisfactorily?
Will it increase our efficiency?
Will it help us meet our targets?
Will this enhance our reputation?

Facilitator/tutor
Did the participants react positively to the
IPE and gain new insights or skills?
Was the preparation, delivery and
evaluation commitment manageable?
What did I learn?

Figure 2.2 Perspectives on the effectiveness of interprofessional education (IPE).

Stakeholders looking at interprofessional education with different eyes are likely to be interested in different outcomes. Recognising this need not become a hopeless case of trying (and failing) to 'please all of the people all of the time'. Fortunately, some perspectives on effective interprofessional education are complementary. Where there is conflict or competition it is helpful to clarify the nature of tensions, enabling appropriate planning, negotiation and compromise.

Figure 2.2 shows some of the ways in which interprofessional education might be effective. For example, in delivering particular outcomes and justifying or streamlining the use of resources. Focusing on outcomes and synthesising reports from over 200 evaluations of interprofessional education (Freeth *et al.* 2002), we concluded that well planned and delivered interprofessional education can produce positive outcomes that can be categorised using a modified form of the four-level Kirkpatrick typology. Our six-fold typology is shown in Table 2.1. The outcome levels are not hierarchical. Each may be sought from any interprofessional education initiative.

Boxes 12.1 to 12.6 in Section III are examples of evaluations of interprofessional education that found changes at each of the levels in Table 2.1.

At level 1 interprofessional education has been effective if participants become (or remain) well disposed towards learning with, from and about other professionals. They might perceive that they have gained insights or knowledge through interprofessional learning that will improve the care they subsequently offer. They may simply feel the educational experience was more stimulating and its content more memorable because of its interactive nature and the diversity of the participants. Effective interprofessional education would avoid negative reactions, whether these emanated from the interprofessional nature of the event or other facets of the interprofessional experience. This amounts to a double responsibility. Inadequate facilities, uninspiring learning resources or poor quality facilitation generate negative learner reactions throughout education.

Table 2.1 Typology for outcomes of interprofessional education.

1	Reaction	Learners' views on the learning experience and its interprofessional nature
2a	Modification of attitudes/perceptions	Changes in reciprocal attitudes or perceptions between participant groups. Changes in perception or attitude towards the value and/or use of team approaches to caring for a specific client group
2b	Acquisition of knowledge/skills	Including knowledge and skills linked to interprofessional collaboration
3	Behavioural change	Identifies individuals' transfer of interprofessional learning to their practice setting and changed professional practice
4a	Change in organisational practice	Wider changes in the organisation and delivery of care
4b	Benefits to patients/clients, families and communities	Improvements in health or well-being of patients/clients, families and communities

In interprofessional education there is a risk that these facets of an unsatisfactory learning experience become, in the minds of the participants, associated with interprofessional collaboration.

To prevent negative reactions, interprofessional education must first and foremost be high quality *education*. Then there should be some added value from its interprofessional nature. Adding this value is demanding. Many of you reading this know all about that. It means, amongst other things, challenging tradition and introducing innovation. Staff working in these ways know well the struggles and costs involved in such work. Without this added value interprofessional education is mere political correctness.

Effective interprofessional education can produce positive cognitive and behavioural changes. At level 2a interprofessional education has been effective if attitudes and perceptions have become more positive, while at level 2b effectiveness requires an increase in knowledge or skill. These attributes are distinguished in the outcomes typology, for practical purposes. Assigning them to different places is not a judgement on their importance. Each is an essential component of learning to be interprofessional.

The positive changes at levels 2a and 2b will hopefully lead to positive behavioural changes (level 3). This is a pivotal point and difficult to achieve. Here the effectiveness of interprofessional education is contingent on overcoming resistance to change within the individual, and amongst their colleagues and clients, and in relation to organisational structures. This may be easier with work-based interprofessional education, involving naturally occurring teams, but this may cause problems for simultaneously continuing to deliver care. Another approach is to involve a critical mass of those working in a particular area, or to systematically build a critical mass. Pre-qualification interprofessional education may be seen as a contribution to this (see for example Boxes 1.2 and 1.5).

Ultimately, for interprofessional education to be deemed effective, patients and clients, families and communities must benefit in some way or another. This might be more seamless care (level 4a as shown in Box 12.5), or safer care with greater efficacy (level 4b as shown in Box 12.6).

Measuring and judging the effectiveness of interprofessional education

In Section III we will focus on the evaluation of interprofessional education in some detail. Here we wish to herald some important questions that are further developed there. For now, we invite you reflect on these questions in conjunction with Figure 2.2, preferably the version that you previously expanded to include your local stakeholders.

- Who measures the effectiveness of interprofessional education and who should measure it?

- Who judges the effectiveness of interprofessional education and who should judge it?
- Why is it difficult to establish the effectiveness of education? Is it especially difficult to do so for interprofessional education?

Improving the effectiveness of interprofessional education

Teaching and learning, the key elements of education, are not independent. The processes of planning, delivering and receiving knowledge are inextricably linked to the teachers and learners involved. In most cases a wider group of people also contribute, for example course administrators and funding managers. In addition to the variable human element of interprofessional education, there is a physical and organisational context that will play its part in the effectiveness of the programme or event. All interact to influence the effectiveness of an interprofessional initiative.

Thinking about improving effectiveness can help you to identify possibilities and choices. It aids strategic planning and emphasises the situated nature of each interprofessional education initiative. One size fits all simply isn't an option. Your interprofessional education course will have unique features that determine what effectiveness model will work best. Consider what lies within your control. Allow yourself to be creative and ambitious in this. The next question is: which changes would be most effective? How might these be set in motion? Who is responsible or capable of doing this? In what order should these changes be made? And so on. We return to this complexity in Sections II and III, in particular in our discussion of the 3P curriculum model for interprofessional education.

Conclusion

In this chapter we have argued that the issues and challenges of measuring the effectiveness of interprofessional education need to be viewed from two perspectives. First, the context in which this type of learning takes places and, second, the forces that act upon and influence its delivery. We have shown that the health and social care context is one in which the measurement of performance is often prioritised, oversimplified and can be burdensome to practitioners in a given education or clinical service setting. Opposing forces act upon the education being delivered in these circumstances. Taking control, with a view to making changes to these forces and thus enhancing effectiveness, is demanding. Nevertheless, finding out about and improving the effectiveness of an interprofessional education initiative is a professional responsibility. In health and social care settings this embraces the impact of the educational initiative for the learner and the impact at the point of delivery of care.

Key points

- Effective interprofessional education means delivering positive outcomes, at acceptable cost, without unacceptable side effects.
- Effectiveness is about what is actually achieved within the complexity of the real world.
- Effectiveness is a multifaceted and contestable concept.
- Effectiveness measures work best when they take account of the context of an initiative and the forces at work within that context.

Further reading

Brennan, J. & Shah, T. (2000) *Managing Quality in Higher Education, an International Perspective on Institutional Assessment and Change.* OECD, SRHE, Open University Press, Buckingham. (Particularly Introduction pp. 1–8 and Quality assessment in higher education: a conceptual model pp. 9–18.)

Degeling, P., Maxwell, S., Iedema, R. & Hunter, D.J. (2004) Making clinical governance work. *British Medical Journal,* **329,** 679–81.

Dewar, S. (2000) Collaborating for quality: the need to strengthen accountability. *Journal of Interprofessional Care,* **14** (1), 31–8.

Jackson, S. (1998) Organisational effectiveness within National Health Service (NHS) trusts. *International Journal of Health Care Quality Assurance,* **11** (6/7), 216–21.

Perkins, R. (2001) What constitutes success? The relative priority of service users' and clinicians' views of mental health services. *British Journal of Psychiatry,* **179,** 9–10.

Swage, T. (2003) *Clinical Governance in Health Care Practice.* 2nd edn. Butterworth-Heinemann, Oxford.

Watts, C. (2000) Issues of professionalism in higher education. In: *New Directions in Professional Higher Education* (eds T. Bourner, T. Katz & D. Watson), pp. 11–18. SRHE and Open University Press, Buckingham.

Useful websites

www.bemecollaboration.org
www.campbellcollaboration.org
www.cochrane.org
www.eppi.ioe.ac.uk

Section II
Developing Effective Interprofessional Education

Introduction

Ideally, development, approval, delivery and evaluation are integrated parts of an iterative process. Taking that as the model, development is evolutionary and continuous. Approval recognises the need for some flexibility in the curriculum and delivery involves being alert to new policies and practices on behalf of the students. In the same way, formative evaluation is just as important as summative evaluation, processes as important as outcomes.

In Section II of this book we take the theoretical models of interprofessional education and effectiveness forward. This means getting to grips with the practical reality of developing a learning experience for two or more health and social care practitioners that enables them to learn with, from and about each other. Chapter three highlights ways towards achieving equilibrium between interprofessional, multi-professional and uni-professional education. Groundwork and curriculum development, and teaching and learning interprofessionally, are the focus of attention in Chapters four to six and in Chapter seven we concentrate on professional development issues. Finally, in Chapter eight we discuss accreditation.

Our views on developing effective interprofessional education have been shaped by reading and experience of course development, in a variety of contexts, with all the ups and downs naturally associated with this type of work. We share these with you as a series of case studies and continue to refer to them during our commentary on evaluation in Section III.

First, we want to present a short commentary on the concept of curriculum. We are introducing this term for efficiency in subsequent chapters, not to overcomplicate the main messages of this book. The concept of curriculum will be used as a mechanism to enable a shared understanding of the multiple elements that need consideration in order that an education or training proposal translates from a good idea to an effective experience. Our intention is to prepare for the chapters in Section II by highlighting the diverse nature of curricula and their crucial importance to the work of establishing effective education. You may want to return to this section during the detailed development of your course.

The curriculum conceptualised

In this book we use the word curriculum as an overarching term for all those aspects of education that contribute to the experience of learning: aims, content, mode of delivery, assessment, and so on. As the book progresses we will look closely at many of these and discuss their contribution to educational effectiveness. The multifaceted concept of curriculum is a useful way of understanding events that are planned with the intention that learning takes place, for example, events within the visible spectrum of interprofessional education introduced in Chapter one and depicted in Figures 1.1 to 1.3.

The notion of curriculum embraces a wide range of models. Problem and enquiry-based learning are examples where small group work is essential to the learning process. Information technology is a key component of web-based curricula for either individuals or small groups. Learner-led curricula, using mechanisms such as personal professional development plans, are increasingly utilised within continued professional development initiatives. All these, and more, have a legitimate place in a number of different planned learning initiatives.

If the term curriculum sounds too grand for a small-scale interprofessional staff development workshop, please think again. Our view is that all planned learning experiences have a curriculum and each curriculum has the following features in some form or another:

- A statement of what the education event hopes to achieve. This may be made public as listed learning outcomes, or course aims and/or objectives, or it may reside mainly in the head of the lead curriculum developer. Potential dangers of this are obvious.
- The rationale for the education event, why it is necessary, its role in respect of current policy and practice and how it fits with local service and organisational need.
- A syllabus, or list of topics to be covered during the course or event. This is often referred to as the course content.
- A teaching strategy or plan, to include teaching methods. This may be underpinned by an explicit educational philosophy such as problem-based learning or a plan-do-study-act quality improvement cycle; or arise from traditional pedagogic custom and practice.
- An assessment strategy or plan, to include the timing, nature and frequency of formative and summative assessments. Written examinations, coursework and placement reports are all legitimate ways of doing this. Self assessment is included in this, for example comments on whether participants' expectations of learning have been met through a short course or during a quality improvement team meeting.
- Resource statements: human, financial, technological, estates, etc.

May we suggest that you now take a few moments to think about your own interprofessional education initiative using the concept of curriculum? What are its main facets? How explicit are these for you and for other stakeholders? How are curriculum decisions made, implemented and evaluated? Who makes these decisions? In what ways could clearer thinking about curriculum help you to develop and deliver effective interprofessional education?

One way of dividing up the features of a curriculum is to separate those that focus on:

- The processes involved in realising the aims and objectives of the course, for example the teaching and learning methods

and

- The content most often found in the syllabus, but also reflected in reading lists and through the key texts and policy documents cited in the rationale given for the event

Arguably, process is more important in interprofessional education than content. The content can be delivered to uni-professional groups of learners, but interprofessional education has been chosen with the added value of interactive learning. The content of interprofessional education, just like the content of all education, will inevitably date. The essential outcome is the development of transferable skills relevant to collaboration and teamwork skills, such as problem solving, and initiating and improving care and the embedding of these in practice.

For pre-qualification interprofessional education, process-focused educators would favour learning and teaching methods that gave students some insight into the reality of working together. These include problem-based learning, interprofessional practice placements, or simulations of aspects of professional practice. Similarly, post-qualification interprofessional education developers might favour work-based learning through quality improvement cycles and action-learning sets. At both levels these relatively challenging methods of teaching and learning are widely supplemented (or substituted) with more traditional workshops that include interprofessional discussion.

Content is nevertheless important. Certain content has to be learnt (and subsequently updated) to permit the delivery of safe and effective care. Policies of the statutory bodies that govern health and social work practice frequently determine much of this type of content, designating it essential for a named professional award. Content also provides motivation to learn, by filling recognised gaps in the learners' knowledge, or by capturing their imaginations and harnessing the energy of this enthusiasm. This means that content should be relevant to learners' concerns and professional practice. Recalling the section on the uniqueness of interprofessional education at the end of Chapter one, interprofessional education requires content to be relevant to the learning needs and interests of a diverse group. This presents challenges. There is a need for careful planning and recognition of staff development needs. We will pick up these threads in Chapters five and seven. In addition, the nature of interprofessional education increases the likelihood that content is contested. Curriculum developers, tutors and learners from different professions or different academic schools will all initially want material that is familiar and pertinent to their particular perspective. We will continue this thread in Chapter six.

Facets of curriculum: planned, delivered, received and hidden

All planned education has a curriculum. Inevitably, the curriculum is more concrete for structured and longer programmes of study than it is for intermittent learning experiences in the workplace. Formal courses are normally well (some may say too well) documented. However, a few moments inspection of, for example, a plan-do-study-act initiative will bring elements of curriculum into view. There will be aims, a rationale, some content, chosen learning processes and resource statements.

Besides recognising these components of curriculum it is important to note that, just as we discussed in relation to effectiveness in Chapter two, the curriculum can be conceived in different ways. These are summarised in Table 2. As we will explain later, it is valuable to have these in mind as you plan your interprofessional education. For the moment we wish to draw particular attention to the hidden curriculum or unplanned learning, as these are often not immediately recognised.

Table 2   Different conceptions of the curriculum.

Planned curriculum	Also known as the curriculum in theory, this is the agreed education package that is anticipated to achieve the desired learning by participants. It may be set out in course documentation and a student handbook.
Delivered curriculum	The curriculum from the perspective of the tutors or trainers, once the planned education 'goes live', and becomes a concrete experience for tutors and learners.
Received curriculum – formal	The curriculum from the perspective of learners during the timetabled activities, e.g. lectures and action-learning sets.
Received curriculum – informal	The curriculum from the perspective of learners during non-timetabled activities of the course, e.g. coffee break discussions and student initiated additional work.
Hidden curriculum	Also called covert learning, this encompasses unplanned learning not readily or immediately recognised. Recognition may occur at a later date but not necessarily. In here is what we learn from the experience of being. This often leads to behavioural changes but may remain unacknowledged as the reason for the change.

You may recall that the hidden curriculum was located within the barely visible encircling bands of learning in Figure 1.2 as we elaborated our model of interprofessional education in Chapter one.

The learning outcomes of the hidden curriculum may be positive, neutral or negative. It is its negative manifestations that usually give rise to concern. For example, students may 'learn' that your educational initiative is not central to their professional development because it is not assessed (or at post-qualification level not awarded continuing professional development credit) while all other components of their professional education are assessed or yield continuous professional development points. Or participants might 'learn' that interprofessional collaboration is little more than politically correct rhetoric. The drivers supporting this malign hidden curriculum could include a lack of resource allocation relative to other aspects of professional education. This difference can make it difficult for learners to attend, or for a satisfactory learning experience to be provided. If those who provide the interprofessional education demonstrate through their behaviour and expressed attitudes a lack of commitment to interprofessional or inter-agency collaboration then this will provide a negative role model for the learners.

Looking for outcomes of the hidden curriculum is important, particularly if they contradict the formal, explicit outcomes of the planned education. You may be able to work out from investigation of the outcomes the processes that cause them. These processes may be amenable to change, improving the overall quality of your educational initiative.

We discuss different approaches to the curriculum in Chapter five. If you want to find out more about different curriculum models, their advantages and disadvantages take a look at the list of suggested further reading.

Key points

- Curriculum is an overarching term for all those aspects of education that contribute to the experience of learning
- All planned learning experiences have a curriculum
- Features of a curriculum can be divided into those that focus on the process and the content
- Different facets of curriculum include those that are planned, delivered, received and hidden

Further reading

Allan, J. (1996) Learning outcomes in higher education. *Studies in Higher Education* **21** (1), 93–108.

Barnett, R., Parry, G. & Coate, K. (2001) Conceptualising curriculum change. *Teaching in Higher Education*, **6** (4), 435–49.

Bell, R., Johnson, K. & Scott, H. (1997) Interprofessional education and curriculum development: a model for the future. In: *Community Health Care Development* (ed. D. Hennessy), pp. 123–58 PalgraveMacMillan, London.

Curry, L. & Wergin, J. F. (1993) *Educating Professionals. Responding to New Expectations for Competence and Accountability*. Jossey-Bass, San Francisco.

Harden, R.M. (1998) *Approaches to Curriculum Planning: ASME Medical Education Booklet 21*. ASME, Edinburgh.

Harden, R.M. (1999) *Ten Questions to Ask when Planning a Course or Curriculum: ASME Medical Education Booklet 20*. ASME, Edinburgh.

Miller, J., Bligh, J., Stanley, I. & Al-Shehri, A. (1998) Motivation and continuation of professional development. *British Journal of General Practice*, **48**, 1429–32.

Whitston, K. (1998) Key skills and curriculum reform. *Studies in Higher Education*, **23** (3), 307–319.

3 Towards Equilibrium

In this chapter we set out the need for achieving equilibrium in choices that involve interprofessional education. A curriculum model is suggested as the means towards the ends of assessing and balancing the influences on interprofessional education initiatives.

Terminology

More than a decade ago Leathard (1994, p. 5) wrote about the 'semantic quagmire' that surrounded interprofessional education. She listed an array of prefixes (inter-, multi-), adjectives (professional, disciplinary) and nouns (education, training) that were used to describe interprofessional education. Today people continue to use a variety of terms such as 'multiprofessional education', 'joint learning', 'shared training', 'interdisciplinary education' and 'common learning', sometimes interchangeably, sometimes with clear separate definitions, and sometimes to obfuscate.

We will not dwell on this, except to say that it is wise to be tolerant of such terminological promiscuity. Being open to the words others may use to describe interprofessional education widens the experiences and expertise that can be drawn upon in your own work. However, the bewildering range of terms in this area, and their inconsistent use, also provides opportunities for confusion, miscommunication and unmatched expectations. It is important to clarify your own thinking when you choose particular terms, but also not to assume that others will interpret those terms in the same way. This can be an important part of the process of developing effective interprofessional education (see Chapters four and five).

For clarity we will reiterate from Chapter one the definitions of interprofessional education and multi-professional education that we use in this book, adding a definition for uni-professional education. These are displayed in Table 3.1. Here we refer to the health and social care professions and it is those in particular that inform the review work (reported in our companion volume *Effective Interprofessional Education: Argument, Assumption and Evidence*, Barr *et al.*, 2005) that this book draws on. We also recognise the contribution of other professionals in achieving health and well-being for people, families and communities, including practitioners of law, architecture and religion, voluntary sector workers and volunteers, elected community leaders, and many more.

Table 3.1 Key definitions.

Interprofessional education/training (IPE) Members (or students) of two or more professions associated with health or social care, engaged in learning *with, from* and *about* each other. It is an initiative to secure interprofessional learning and promote gains through interprofessional collaboration in professional practice.

Multi-professional education (MPE) Members (or students) of two or more professions learning alongside one another: parallel learning rather than interactive learning.

Uni-professional education Members (or students) of a single profession learning together: interactively or in parallel.

We acknowledge that uni-professional education is an unattractive phrase, but within this book subtle distinctions need to be made. It is not sufficient to use the term professional education. This would imply that interprofessional education and multi-professional education are separate from professional education rather than integral parts of it. Interprofessional education, multi-professional education and uni-professional education can together make up a 'whole'. This leads into the main focus of this chapter: selecting an effective balance between interprofessional, multi-professional and uni-professional education (see also Barr *et al.*, 2005).

Selecting an effective balance of interprofessional, multi-professional and uni-professional education

Interprofessional education and uni-professional education complement one another, each helping practitioners to develop or update the knowledge, skills and attitudes they require for effective professional practice. Interprofessional and inter-agency work is part of professional work. It is essential that both types of education prepare practitioners so that they recognise when collaboration is necessary, and when the responsibility for an aspect of care is solely theirs.

Uni-professional education will focus on the learning needs of one profession. Much of this will be profession-specific knowledge and skills, but uni-professional education should not ignore developing competencies for interprofessional and inter-agency collaboration as a learning need for every health and social care professional. Recognition of a duty to collaborate effectively on behalf of clients and patients should become embedded in professional thinking as a result of learning experiences across the curriculum. This can be achieved through, for example, case management exercises, observing the practice of more experienced colleagues, and threads running through every part of a programme addressing a patient focus and empowering clients, communication, ethical practice and effective care.

Interprofessional education will be employed where the interaction between members (or students) of a number of professions is essential for the planned learning (see for example Boxes 1.3 and 1.4); or adds value to the planned learning to an extent that justifies any additional resource required for interprofessional education (see for example Box 1.5). Naturally, in cases where interprofessional education offers resource savings over uni-professional education, interprofessional education will be preferred, but we have not yet located an example of this type. Indeed, in Chapter two we noted that interprofessional education can be judged as relatively expensive at the point of delivery, due to the need for group sizes small enough to facilitate effective interaction. Travel costs and more complex administration are added extras where students from different courses attend from different home sites.

Multi-professional education, on some occasions, may make a useful contribution to the efficient use of resources. It may permit certain professional groups to benefit from learning opportunities that they would otherwise be denied. Box 3.1 is an example of this. However, we would encourage attention to the interaction necessary to convert multi-professional education into interprofessional education, thereby adding value to the learning and promoting collaborative practice.

Most professional education will probably always be uni-professional, with proportions of multi-professional and interprofessional according to the needs

---

Box 3.1 A multi-professional anatomy module.

Mitchell *et al.* (2004) describe an evaluation of a multi-professional anatomy module for biomedical science, medicine, nursing, physiotherapy, diagnostic radiography and therapeutic radiography students. Students attended anatomy classes in a dissecting room in small mixed groups, over a series of weeks. Each group observed the dissection of a cadaver by a trained demonstrator. During the dissection process students focused on basic anatomy of the skeletal, muscular, nervous, cardiovascular, respiratory, digestive and urogenital systems.

Each student was given a handbook with instructions on each session's learning outcomes and was expected to use this as a guide to answering a series of questions related to the cadaver. They also took a clinical skills teaching session, in which issues related to anatomy were linked to appropriate clinical examination skills. All students completed an end-of-course assessment of 40 questions on anatomy.

A post-course evaluation of questionnaire responses from the students indicated that the majority of them enjoyed their multi-professional learning experience. Student assessment results varied widely, with the medical and physiotherapy students recording the highest scores.

The authors conclude that a multi-professional approach to teaching anatomy is feasible. However, an over-emphasis on medicine during the anatomy sessions needed amendment to ensure that nursing, diagnostic radiography and therapeutic radiography students' assessment scores could match those of the medical and physiotherapy students.

of particular target learners or particular content. We believe that all professional education should contain a thread of interprofessional education, whose emphasis should vary according to educational need. From time to time there may be sufficient educational justification for the provision of a small element of multiprofessional education.

Finding the optimum balance between interprofessional and uni-professional education has no certain answers. Neither are there any direct means of enumeration on either side of the equation. Balance could be measured in terms of timing, frequency or total time allocated; or the proportion of tutor time, learning resources and classroom space allocated; or the balance of assessment, and so on. However, the important balance is that of impact on subsequent professional practice. Striving for balance should be seen as a continuing journey, starting within today's constraints and working towards an ever more effective balance of 'joined up' interprofessional and uni-professional education. One day, maybe, it will be seamless.

An effective balance between interprofessional and uni-professional education helps to develop and maintain effective interprofessional care. It aims to provide participants with the knowledge and motivation necessary to evaluate success and, where appropriate, to strive for improvement.

In planning for effective balance within and between education initiatives for health and social care practitioners we see education as a diverse range of means and ends to secure learning. It is this learning that enables and influences people to provide high quality care within resource constraints. Thinking broadly, not restricting opportunities for interprofessional education to any particular service setting, academic level, or designated groups of practitioners, is the way towards this (see also Barr *et al.* 2005).

Presage, process and product

Briefly, we would like to introduce a curriculum model that may help you to achieve equilibrium between your interprofessional education and the wider curriculum. The model is a means of seeking balance within interprofessional education and we refer back to it in subsequent chapters. Two of us have discussed elsewhere the usefulness of this curriculum model for informing decisions about the management, development and delivery of interprofessional education (Freeth & Reeves, 2004).

The 3P (presage-process-product) model of learning and teaching was first elaborated as a system by Biggs (1993). It is a useful device for structuring discussion of the components and dynamics of planned educational experiences and we have elaborated it in the context of interprofessional education (Figure 3.1). Biggs' form of the model included our central presage box as part of the context for learning and teaching element. We have chosen to highlight the

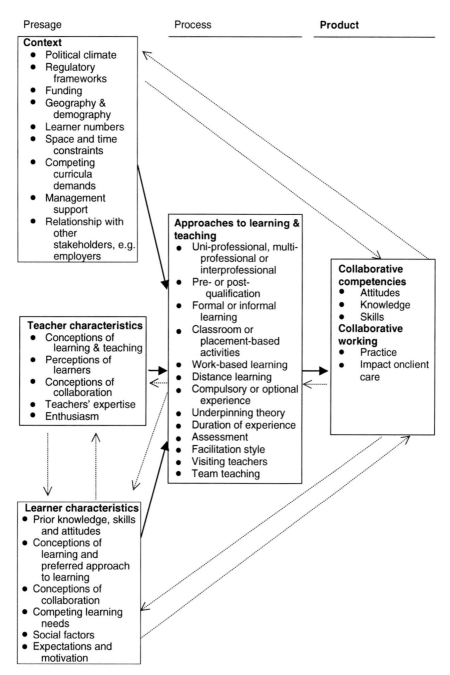

Figure 3.1 The 3P model related to interprofessional education. Adapted from Freeth & Reeves (2004).

importance of the people that shape and deliver professional education by treating their influences as a separate strand of presage factors.

Presage factors include constraints and opportunities, such as requirements for professional registration, funding, tutors' expertise and enthusiasm, participants' prior learning and beliefs. Process factors include the selection of particular approaches to learning and teaching, the balance between workplace and classroom learning, whether the interprofessional learning is optional or compulsory. These lists are not exhaustive. Products include collaborative competencies and attitudes, knowledge, skills and actions in practice that reflect the focus of the course content. In addition, as a result of the hidden curriculum (see note in the introduction to Section II), there may be unintended and possibly undesirable outcomes.

There is a natural flow from left to right in Figure 3.1. Presage factors exist before the learning experience. They influence the creation, conduct and outcomes of learning experiences. Process factors describe a particular learning and teaching mix. They lead to the product or outcomes of learning. However, it is too simplistic to assume that knowledge of presage will permit the manipulation of process to produce the desired outcomes. As the arrows in Figure 3.1 indicate, the 3P model represents a complex and dynamic system. Some presage factors influence the product directly. Presage factors interact with each other. Feedback occurs at all stages of the model. The curriculum as a dynamic system seeks equilibrium.

We suggest that greater analysis of presage, process and product in relation to interprofessional education would be beneficial. This analysis needs to be conducted by those who commission interprofessional education; and those who develop and deliver it. Some of the influencing factors lie largely within their control. Others must be accommodated. The 3P model enables structured evaluation of creative responses to genuine constraints. In addition, assumed immutability can be challenged, areas for improvement can be identified, and the likely consequences of proposed innovation can be explored. This critical analysis of possibilities, together with explicit recognition of decision-making processes, will contribute to better-targeted management of educational processes.

We will return to the 3P model in the next chapter, sketching out some of the detail of its components. For now, let us return to the spectrum of interprofessional education described in Chapter one, for example Figure 1.1. This has been reproduced and elaborated as Figure 3.2. Balancing the processes and content of interprofessional education occurs through balancing presage factors (some of which are shown in Figure 3.2) and taking control of educational processes within your interprofessional education. The joint outcome of the balancing and proactive creation of learning opportunities dictates where your interprofessional education lies within the progressively shaded rectangle.

The next section will provide some questions that may help you to consider matters of presage and process in your own context, helping you to challenge presage and refine process so that your desired products (outcomes) become a reality.

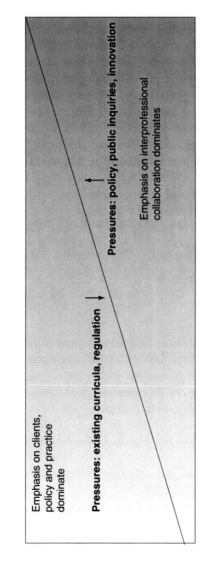

Figure 3.2 Pressures balancing the content of interprofessional education.

Questions supporting decisions on effective balance

There are several important questions related to identifying the balance that you aim to provide in relation to your interprofessional education development. Reflecting upon presage and process need not be confined to the pre-delivery stages of a learning experience. It is equally useful as part of an evaluation. We will discuss this further in Section III. It can also be used as a 'reality check' during more ad hoc and opportunistic interprofessional learning that takes place in the reality of the workplace without an explicit educational plan, often associated with quality assurance, audit, or clinical governance. This may be especially, but not exclusively, helpful if the process did not achieve as much as had been hoped for.

The following list is given for you to reflect upon in relation to your own context. It is not exhaustive. Add others that are important to your own situation. Each major question leads into subsidiary questions to prompt your thinking.

- Who chooses the balance of what is delivered?
    - Who should be making these choices?
    - What is the effect of placing these choices with these people or at these levels?

- Do I have an active choice here?
    - Have the choices already been made by others that I can no longer influence?

- How can this interprofessional education fit within a coherent whole?
    - How can I avoid my interprofessional education being a 'bolt-on' extra?
    - How can I minimise overloading learners and tutors?
    - What, if anything, can be removed from the present curriculum to make space for interprofessional learning?

- What will be the effects of the planned interprofessional education on the rest of the curriculum?
    - Will there be duplication of effort, economies of scale and opportunities for exciting new projects?
    - What are the requirements for revisions elsewhere to ensure a good fit between interprofessional and other learning?
    - What is the balance of gains and losses?
    - What will be the nature and impact of the losses?
    - Who is likely to mourn these losses and how destructive could this process be?

- When should this interprofessional education occur?
    - How does it fit into the other parts of the learning process?

- What about its duration and frequency?
- Where should it take place?

- How many stakeholders can I deal with effectively at this stage?
  - Would it be better to go for wholesale redevelopment of several programmes of learning to maximise the possibility of lasting structural and cultural change?
  - Would it be better to demonstrate success with a small number of people within existing frameworks and hope that success encourages expansion and embedding of the initiative?

Conclusion

This chapter has discussed the choices available to you during the process of developing an interprofessional education initiative. We have introduced and elaborated upon the notion of curriculum and identified one curriculum model in particular. All this sets the scene for our subsequent discussion on the practice of curriculum development, the choices made and the decision-making processes that contribute to the end product. Your deliberations are just the beginning of a long journey. How to prepare the ground for that journey and signposts along the way are mapped out in the following chapters.

Key points

- Interprofessional education has a clear focus on *interaction* between participating professionals
- Interprofessional education and uni-professional education complement one another and each contributes to effective professional practice
- Interprofessional curricula are dynamic systems that seek equilibrium
- The presage-process-product model of learning is a useful device for structuring discussion of the components and dynamics of planned educational experiences

Further reading

Francis, B. & Humphreys, J. (2000) Professional education as a structural barrier to lifelong learning in the NHS. *Journal of Education Policy*, **15** (3), 281–92.
Freeth, D. & Reeves, S. (2003) Learning to work together: using the presage, process, product (3P) model to highlight decisions and possibilities. *Journal of Interprofessional Care*, **18** (1), 43–56.

Harden, R. M. (1998) Effective multi-professional education: a three-dimensional perspective. AMEE guide 12: multi-professional education: part 1. *Medical Teacher*, **20** (5), 402–408.

Hurst, K. (1999) Educational implications of multiskilled health carers. *Medical Teacher*, **21** (2), 170–73.

Pirrie, A. (1999) Rocky Mountains and tired Indians: on territories and tribes. Reflections on multidisciplinary education in the health professions. *British Educational Research Journal*, **25** (1), 113–26.

Woodcock, A., White, P., Smith, H., Coles, C., Campion-Smith, C. & Stannard, T. (2000) GP selection of postgraduate courses has implications for colleagues: messages for course providers and for those writing practice developmental plans. *British Journal of General Practice*, **50**, 785–790.

4 The Groundwork

In this chapter we look at the political climate that surrounds the development of an interprofessional education initiative, from the perspective of institutional and personal relationships. The emphasis is on what can be done in preparation for the demanding work of course planning and the factors that influence the success of that work.

Introduction

The groundwork discussed in this chapter refers to what needs to be done before the development of an interprofessional education initiative. We have called this preparatory work *planning* and those involved in it *the planning team*. This may, or may not, be the same group of people who take the work forward into course development. We will refer to this group as the *development team* and we focus on their work mostly in Chapter five. Some of the comments we make here apply to both teams and then we simply use the word *team*.

The planning team will vary in its membership depending on the nature of the education to be developed. For a short training course there may not be a planning team: one person may take on the responsibility for getting the development team together. It would, of course, be contrary to the principles of interprofessional education if this lone individual then took the initiative forward. Developing interprofessional education is a collaborative task. Input from colleagues who share perspectives with the potential learners is fundamentally important to the final shape and success of the course. For many initiatives, planning will be the responsibility of a group of people. Some may continue to work on the development of the education: others may be better placed to participate in a consultative role, perhaps becoming part of a longer-term steering group for complex programmes of study that continue over several years.

You may be thinking that all this seems unnecessarily complicated. For some interprofessional initiatives, for example a half-day in-service training session, this is a fair judgement. In most cases, however, as we show here and later, there is a level of complexity associated with the development of interprofessional education, over and above that linked to education in general. This is one reason why we advocate piloting interprofessional education initiatives, which will be discussed further in Chapter five.

Pilot programmes allow valuable insight into many of the issues that might become hurdles in the way of successfully delivering effective interprofessional education. Hurdles relating to local and professional politics, the diversity of the stakeholders and the need to find common ground about education principles and processes within different professional cultures. Interprofessional teams, during planning and development, often need to work with different financial control systems, at least two, and maybe more, institutional contexts, and in various geographies. Attention to the groundwork can make a substantial difference to achieving your aims and to the effectiveness of the education initiative that results from development work.

The next sections expand on all these issues from two perspectives. We pay attention to how the work of the planning team can be influenced by the strengths and weaknesses of the externalities of which it must take notice. Our focus is also on the internal working of that team and the ways in which, for example, politics and culture, can be played out between its members (see also Barr *et al.*, 2005). Teamworking demands certain skills and the adaptation of *personal* and *usual* practices. When the requirement is for interprofessional teamwork there are further demands. During the planning stage similar relationship factors operate to those that will be apparent in the interprofessional education when it is delivered. The planning team themselves will, in effect, be immersed in interprofessional learning.

Factors that make interprofessional education challenging may not be felt equally throughout the planning team. Institutional and peer pressures vary according to the experience of organisations and professions with interprofessional education. For some it is a very new venture, others may be old hands and willing to participate yet again. There may be those who feel threatened or disheartened by the prospect of being involved with interprofessional education, often those without any experience, but also those with unhappy experience behind them.

An awareness of the issues outlined above and attentiveness to the way they shape the hard work of being involved in interprofessional education can help you along that, sometimes, tortuous pathway. We are wary of sounding too pessimistic here. Our experiences of working interprofessionally have, overall, been very good. But we have learnt lessons and listened to the experiences of colleagues that can be shared. Our aim is to prepare you for the challenges that lie ahead during negotiations with external bodies and those times when the internal teams engage in lively dialogue and debate about the education initiative.

The political arena

All educational development is, in part, a political activity. In other words, it is associated with sets of ideas, principles and commitments. In any organisation, those who hold a particular view on how education should or should not be

delivered may also be in positions of authority in respect to your planned education development. They will be influenced by governmental policies. If these
policies are supportive then they may create the necessary 'incentive' for educational institutions to begin operationalising them. Areskog (1995) argued that
interprofessional education needs to be 'an established part of government policy'
(p. 132) in order to provide the political imperative to successfully establish and
embed it within institutions. In the UK a number of Government policies have
advocated the use of interprofessional education (for example, Department of
Health, 2001). Consequently, there has been an increase in interprofessional
education, but whether this is of the type where learning *with*, *from* and *about*
occurs, bears close examination. For example, Miller *et al.* (1999) found that most
of the shared learning initiatives reported in their survey did not have high
quality interprofessional interaction as a central feature. Most were essentially
multi-professional education initiatives.

Securing sufficient resources

Whether the education initiative is to take place in a clinical setting or classroom
the participating organisations (probably universities and service providers) will
have a stake in your venture. A vital issue is the deployment of resources to
support the interprofessional education during its development, delivery and
evaluation. The political will of senior managers will need to be translated into
the reality of providing funding, staff and physical resources, for example teaching space. The cost of interprofessional education can span different budgets and
the logistics of joint financial arrangements may prove problematic. For example,
if one partner organisation is to provide learning experiences on behalf of all
partner organisations there may a need to transfer funds to follow the learners.
This may disturb organisations' earlier budgeting; rarely a popular process.
Formal contracts may need to be drawn up.

Securing overall funding from an external source can be the means to resolve
such issues. You might like to consider this option if ensuring funding for your
course is one of the hurdles you are anticipating. It will introduce flexibility and
allow freedom from normal budgetary constraints. But the downside is that
external funding is often only available in the short term, to pump-prime a new
initiative. The mental health module described in Box 1.2 is an example of this.
The participating departments will soon have to look at ways of sustaining the
interprofessional education from their core budgets. Nevertheless, in the example
in Box 1.2, vital and expensive development was supported by the external grant,
providing a firm foundation for its continuation.

So, if a course developed with external funds is to continue, permanent and
adequate funding will need to be secured from a substantive institutional
budget(s). Applying for continuing funding after the course has been run once
or twice gives you the advantage of evidence to support your application. This, of
course, reinforces why you should take a sound approach to evaluating the
impact of the course, which will be discussed in Section III.

Funding for interprofessional education needs to take into account the nature of interactive learning, such as small student groups supported by facilitators or high quality self-directed learning resources. Yes, a shared lecture between different professions is less expensive and will achieve economies of scale, but simply sitting people together is unlikely to develop the attitudes or knowledge needed for effective collaboration. Interaction is required to ensure that learners talk, listen, debate, clarify and negotiate with one another: these are key dimensions of effective collaboration. It is your task to convince those holding the purse strings of the necessity and value of the investment requested to support interprofessional learning.

Try to begin the process of negotiating for these resources at an early stage and do not take for granted that assurances of support will automatically be translated into reality. Continuously briefing your senior colleagues on the progress of your development will help to minimise the risk of a funding crisis. Never just assume you have the continued support of the institutions involved. Changes in the health and social care sector and higher education funding priorities happen with alarming frequency; and new initiatives in education can be seen as something that can be put on hold, or even permanently displaced, by apparently more urgent short-term needs.

You will need to learn about the processes of interaction and negotiation that are involved in securing funding and other support in your local context. It can be important to identify who has the authority to act on behalf of each participating institution on a variety of matters; and the limits of their authority. For example, a promise of rooms is only that until the department that allocates teaching space puts your course into their timetabling system. We advise seeking written assurances and, where necessary, inter-institutional contracts.

The role of champions

Champions who help to persuade others to support an interprofessional education initiative are very important people. Two of the ways they can be helpful are speaking in favour of proposals at decision-making meetings and influencing the staff in their teams and areas of practice to be positively disposed to the interprofessional education. They may make resources available or alert the planning team to the availability of resources elsewhere. Such people are also often able to give advance warning of political or organisational changes that might be predicted to influence the implementation of interprofessional education.

There are natural and long-term champions for interprofessional education who will tend to advocate its role as opportunities arise throughout their careers, those with the experience to support a firm conviction that interprofessional education leads to joined-up working and improved care. Others may be more strategic champions of interprofessional education. Sometimes they are driven by the realisation that supporting and being involved with a politically valued initiative is not only good for their institution but also for their career. Then again there are passionate champions with a short attention span; people who crave the variety of moving from one interesting and good idea to the next. In the development of the interprofessional initiative described in Box 1.3, an M.Sc. course for those working with survivors of violence, Sully (2002) stressed the important role of champions in successfully bringing together health care professionals, police officers and people from voluntary organisations.

The type of champion you are working with may not matter very much in the short term; all can give valuable drive to the development of interprofessional education. Champions are often promoted or headhunted for other initiatives. If they are highly respected in your context they are probably well respected elsewhere too. If you are unlucky, their new priority will be in direct competition with your current interprofessional education initiative. More often, the movement of champions opens up opportunities for wider networking and collaboration, as they seek to apply learning from their former to their new context.

Sooner or later, you may be that champion. What qualities do you need to undertake this role? We would argue that 'hardiness', the ability to work well and effectively under challenging circumstances, is needed. Whilst it is exciting to undertake a new venture that allows you to extend your horizons and work with colleagues from different professions, the obstacles you will face may be formidable. You might meet scepticism, resistance from colleagues and learners, and you might not have full support from the managers within your institution. At these times a colleague who can lend a sympathetic ear and provide critical support is invaluable.

The interprofessional education planning team

As well as the macro-political level discussed above, ideas, principles and commitment play an important part at the micro or individual level. Members of the planning team and those who will later be associated with developing and delivering the education will, perhaps for the first time, recognise the strength of their own professional politics. The product of the team is dependent upon people working effectively together, being committed to the task and with sufficient time to do the work involved. Overcoming institutional barriers may have been your first task; working with individuals is the second. Neither is ever finished: interprofessionality takes time to develop and it is wise to assume that constant attention must be given to ensure good interprofessional relationships at all levels continue to be good.

The need to obtain commitment from tutors and practitioners involved in developing interprofessional education is acknowledged in many published accounts. Reflecting upon their experience with pre-qualification physiotherapy, physician assistant and dental hygiene students who undertook a 12-week interprofessional initiative working in a community-based clinic, Lary *et al.* (1997) argued that course organisers should seek staff who are committed to interprofessional education to develop and deliver an initiative. Sommer *et al.* (1992)

provided a similar illustration. They found that the success of their interprofessional initiative for medical, physiotherapy, occupational therapy and nursing students was largely dependent on the commitment and enthusiasm of the clinical practitioners, acting as facilitators, to find additional time during their busy working week to deliver the course. And the findings of Cook & Drusin (1995) in relation to an interprofessional initiative for pre-qualification medical and nursing students revealed that its development was inhibited by the scepticism of the tutors about the value of collaborative learning and some embedded negative stereotypical opinions about each other's professions.

You might aim to recruit people to the planning team who are known to be committed to interprofessional education and prepared to devote their time, energy and enthusiasm to overcoming various educational, professional and logistical difficulties. This is certainly an attractive approach and may be a useful starting point, but it will not necessarily fill all the roles that are needed on the planning group. You will need to work with staff from all the partner organisations and ideally the planning group should include people with sufficient seniority or delegated authority to effect change. As such, the team will (normally) contain diverse attitudes to, and knowledge and experience of, interprofessional collaboration. Its members may take time to adjust to the border crossing necessary in interprofessional work. We say more about staff development for interprofessional education in Chapter seven.

Planning interprofessional education is an interprofessional education experience in itself. Effective work by the planning group will depend upon collaboration and interaction. You will be learning *with* staff from other professions and organisations. You will have something to learn *from* their contribution to the planning process and they will from yours. You will learn *about* each other, personally and professionally, and about different and distinctive bodies of knowledge. In the particular context of developing interprofessional education for students or practitioners, members of the planning group will gain insight into different views about what sort of knowledge counts, the choices made by professional groups about how to validate that knowledge and the different ways available to teach the knowledge to others.

Some planning teams struggle to work well together. Commitment may be less than ideal. Members may stick with their set ideas about professional education. Insufficient attention may be paid to fostering collaboration and interaction among the planning group and the team may become dysfunctional. If this has been your experience then it will be difficult to try again. But this may apply to any one of the people on the planning team. Time spent at the beginning learning about the experiences and background of all the planning team members is a good investment for the future of that team. Thinking together about team formation (drawing from an extensive literature on team processes), group dynamics, and means for monitoring group processes within the planning team may feel like a distraction from the business of planning the interprofessional education that others will learn from, but attention to processes within the planning normally represents time well spent. You might consider applying the presage-process-product model we discussed in Chapter three (Figure 3.2) not only to the interprofessional education you are planning but also to the work of the planning team.

Working together with initial ideas for an interprofessional education initiative and maintaining a team approach during the subsequent development and delivery are essential ingredients for a successful outcome. Part of the groundwork for this success is establishing shared thinking about the *process* of planning. What is the timescale for development? How will decisions be made and recorded? How will differences be dealt with? Is the end point of the work formal approval or accreditation of the interprofessional education? To what extent will the mechanisms for approval or accreditation that apply to each partner in the interprofessional initiative dictate processes and outcomes? How will the planning group plan accommodate additions to the team and members' departures?

Working on a collaborative project is often undertaken in addition to a normal workload. This can make attendance at joint planning meetings and keeping to deadlines difficult. These considerations, and larger number of stakeholders involved, make it logical to allow longer for the development of an interprofessional education initiative than might be needed for a similar uni-professional development.

All planning team members will need the opportunity to participate in decisions about who should be involved, how much work each member is likely to be asked to contribute and where and when the planning meetings will take place. It is likely that planning team members and, later, those in the development team, will be from different institutions; work on different sites, even in different towns. In some cases, the distances between those involved in developing the course demand a blended approach to communication. For example, teams from Finnish Polytechnics, developing an e-learning interprofessional module on elderly care, did most of the work of planning the module using the web-based technology that later served the students taking the module (Juntunen & Heikkinen, 2004).

Of course, you do not necessarily need a geographical reason to use alternatives to what can be time-consuming face-to-face meetings. Providing all partners have reasonable means of access, establishing an intranet or Internet site for the planning team is a useful mechanism for sharing draft documents and seeking team members' views. However, information technology facilities are underdeveloped in some settings, and some organisations' systems and policies inhibit or forbid the exchange of documents in this way. It is important that the planning team's means of communication and collaborative development aim not to marginalise the contributions of certain members and certain organisations. Groups that might be particularly vulnerable in this respect include service-user representatives, student representatives and practitioners whose workplaces are not well provided with computers and external connectivity.

However efficient alternative means of communication may be, group processes will be enhanced if at least some (maybe the first and last) of your meetings are 'live'. For physical meetings details as mundane as ensuring that where you meet has adequate car parking and that everyone has a map of the venue can make a big difference to the ambience and productivity. The timing and location of team meetings should not systematically inhibit the participation of particular stakeholders; the easiest ones to overlook being students and service users.

Another essential part of team cohesiveness is keeping to agreed deadlines and other commitments. Among the ways in which the diversity within the planning and development teams will be expressed are different organisational and personal work patterns. These influence how much time members have for their individual contributions and the way they execute their contribution. Not producing things on time and not producing things in the way that others expect are two possible sources of friction within a team. Deadlines and expectations need to be as realistic as possible and this is best achieved through discussion with the entire team. It may feel that involving everyone in the discussion of deadlines and expectations is wasting valuable planning and development time but it can go a long way towards preventing later disappointments, frustrations and even rifts. Formal project management methods can be very helpful, including establishing clear timelines, undertaking risk assessments, and performing critical path analysis. If you want to find out more about such methods searching the World Wide Web would be a good place to start. For example, Manktelow (2003) and Baker & Hunt (2002) have useful information about these and will also give you ideas about the software available if you who want to use the tools electronically.

When an interprofessional education initiative involves several organisations and many professions the teams can become very large. Finding mutually convenient times for meetings becomes almost impossible and identifying a suitable venue may also be difficult. It can be difficult for more reticent individuals to make contributions within a large group. It might be expedient to create smaller working groups drawn from the larger planning team. Subgroups often emerge naturally but however they are formed they need guidance from the wider team on the nature of their task, the limits of their authority. Working groups should report regularly to the whole team to avoid unnecessary conflict, disengagement or duplication of effort.

Teams like this will inevitably pass through the stages of *group development* (Tuckman, 1965), able to *perform* only after they have got to know each other (formed), tested ideas and worked through conflict (stormed) and accepted the interprofessional *norms* of the team. For the planning team, after their preliminary work they will prepare to 'adjourn' (Tuckman & Jensen, 1977) by handing over to the development team (see Chapter five). It is worthwhile repeating something we said at the beginning of the chapter about planning team members moving into other roles connected with the work of developing the interprofessional education. Senior managers may be ideal as members of a later steering group; others may join the curriculum development team. You may know at this stage who will continue to be a champion for the initiative and who will continue to take the role of course tutors.

Planning, developing and delivering interprofessional education means that people with diverse backgrounds and work settings will be working closely together for, quite possibly, several months. Over this time the team process will have good and not-so-good moments. The teams may also come under pressure from institutional changes, new drivers and the ever changing political environment. Internal and external changes may cause a return to the storming stage. Recognising the team's work as innovating and managing change is often helpful here. There are several models for managing change and the diffusion of innovation that might be considered useful in such circumstances. Burnes (2000) in the further reading at the end of this chapter provides a useful overview in this area. Box 4.1 summarises a two-year ethnographic study of a planning team.

Being aware of its own group formation processes will help the team to provide suitable activities, time and facilitation support for the group processes that participants will experience within the eventual interprofessional education.

Membership of the planning team

We have already said a little about membership of the planning team. The team needs members that are enthusiastic about interprofessional collaboration and also needs each partner organisation to be represented. Members need sufficient seniority or delegated authority to make decisions and effect change. Champions may be members of the planning team, but if they are not, a mechanism for keeping them informed about decisions and progress will be very important. In addition, each participating profession should have the opportunity of nominating one or two members for the planning team. This will enable the team to have first-hand input from different professional perspectives and considerably reduces the chance of the planning team inadvertently making decisions that will inhibit the participation of one or more professions' practitioners or students. Professions that have traditionally found it difficult to make their voice heard within the multi-professional team may benefit from nominating two full members who can work together in a mutually supportive fashion.

Box 4.1   Observing the planning process.

Reeves (2005) observed the collaborative process between educational and clinical managers as they developed and delivered an interprofessional education initiative. He found that enthusiasm for interprofessional education facilitated positive group relations and supported the development and delivery of the initiative, but also resulted in a lack of critical analysis amongst members, which resembled the characteristics of groupthink (Janis, 1982). This, Reeves observed, resulted in ambiguity about respective roles, lack of debate between members about the development of the initiative and failure to undertake group maintenance activities, which undermined the quality of members' work together and generated tensions. Reeves also noted that external challenges, notably reorganisation in the hospital where the programme was due to be delivered, undermined the group's collaborative work.

Ideally, the planning team will include student and service-user representatives who can offer different perspectives on learning and care that greatly enhance the interprofessional education. These planning team members are relatively power-less within the organisational settings that host interprofessional education initia-tives. They may feel daunted about speaking at meetings and doubt that they have expertise to offer or skills to contribute. It is good practice never to expect students or service users to be the sole representative of their group within a team of diverse professionals. This may mean appointing two members from each group. Organisational and professional members of the planning team must take responsibility for welcoming students and service users into what may seem a strange environment, ensure their out-of-pocket expenses are met and actively seek their views on the appropriate aspects of the curriculum. It may be decided that students and service users are asked to attend only certain meetings in order to make most efficient use of their time.

Alternative ways of eliciting the insights of students and service users is to access existing forums or to create representative panels. The interprofessional education team might take specific questions to these groups or ask for their views on the draft learning outcomes, content and learning materials.

The planning and development process mirrors the interprofessional education under development. The isolation and burden of responsibility that could be felt by certain lone members of the team will be similarly felt by participants in the interprofessional education who are their profession's lone representative within an interprofessional seminar or problem-based learning group. There is added value in the planning and development processes if the teams can reflect on their experience and feed their learning into the subsequent interprofessional educa-tion. Try to allow time for activities that evaluate team processes and make a commitment to echo the team's learning during subsequent curriculum planning discussions.

Membership of the planning team has another facet beyond the representation of all stakeholders. Belbin (1981) described roles adopted by team members (who might each adopt more than one role) and the effect that the absence of particular roles can have (see also www.belbin.com). If, for example, the group contains several 'plants' and no 'completer' you will generate lots of good ideas but may have difficulty in bringing any one to fruition. Your planning team might consider analysing its strengths and weaknesses from this perspective, partly as a means to get to know one another and partly to guard against some of the pitfalls that are so common within unbalanced groups. The same will apply later on to the develop-ment team.

Pre-qualification interprofessional education

There are very few planning issues that are inherently different for pre-qualifica-tion and post-qualification interprofessional education, but we will highlight some that are pertinent.

Developing pre-qualification courses involves overcoming a number of what Pirrie *et al.* (1998) called internal inhibitors. These include (often substantial) inequalities in the number of students from different professions, geographical isolation from one another, and differences in curricula, which cause timetable clashes. There are also external inhibitors such as agreeing joint financial arrangements (as we discussed above) and securing joint or multiple validation and accreditation, since pre-qualification education, including interprofessional education, must meet the requirements for academic awards and criteria for awarding licences to practice.

Post-qualification interprofessional education

A key aspect of post-qualification interprofessional education is the need to serve practitioners in settings where the service must often be delivered round-the-clock. It is rare for complete practice teams to be able to engage in interprofessional education together; their service delivery commitments and differing working patterns inhibit this. However, planning to embed interprofessional education within quality improvement processes can go some way towards overcoming this difficulty. Pragmatically, most post-qualification interprofessional education is targeted at individuals or pairs from teams, brought together with members of other teams. By repeating interprofessional learning opportunities a critical mass of practitioners in a particular service context may engage with similar development opportunities and begin to review and improve the interprofessional collaboration in their practice setting.

University-led post-qualification interprofessional education may be subject to the same approval requirements for academic award as we noted with pre-qualification interprofessional education, but the professional requirements for a licence to practice are less likely to be a concern. Service-led post-qualification interprofessional education may have quite limited approval requirements. However, most professions have continuing professional development requirements and it is good practice to seek to reward learners' participation with continuing professional development credits where this is possible. The planning team may have to assess the feasibility of awarding these credits for each of the participating professions.

Conclusion

Planning a successful interprofessional education experience depends on recognising the contributions of each stakeholder, alternative theoretical paradigms of knowledge transfer and possibilities for new learning and teaching methods. As the development team takes over the work of the planning team and the interprofessional curriculum becomes more and more of a reality, there is a need to manage the pressures arising from balancing profession-specific learning about providing safe, effective care that is tailored to clients' needs and learning about how to deliver that care as an interprofessional team.

In this chapter we have tried to be pragmatic about the complex work of planning interprofessional education. We have highlighted a number of issues that can lead to this type of initiative 'falling at an early hurdle'. Our intention is neither to deter you nor to lessen your enthusiasm but to forewarn you so that you are forearmed.

Key points

- Often, there is need for some preparatory work before interprofessional curriculum development can take place. This is done by a planning team, who may, or may not, be the same as the curriculum development team.
- The planning and development of an educational initiative is inevitably shaped by the ideas, principles and commitments of those who do this work.
- Those who champion interprofessional education are invaluable allies to those involved in planning and developing interprofessional education.
- An effective planning team needs enthusiastic, representative and committed members who can individually play most of the essential roles within an effective team.

Further reading

Bailey, D. (2002a) Training together: part II: an exploration of the evaluation of a shared learning programme on dual diagnosis for specialist drugs workers and approved social workers. *Social Work Education*, **21** (6, Dec.) 685–99.

Bailey, D. (2002b) Training together: an exploration of a shared learning approach to dual diagnosis training for specialist drugs workers and approved social workers (ASWs). *Social Work Education*, **21** (5, Oct.) 565–81.

Brooks, I. (2002) *Organisational Behaviour: Individuals, Groups and Organisation*. 2nd edn. Prentice Hall, London.

Burnes, B. (2000) *Managing Change a Strategic Approach to Organisational Dynamics*. 3rd edn. Pearson Education, Harlow.

Elwyn, G., Hocking, P., Burtonwood, A., Harry, K. & Turner, A. (2002) Learning to plan? A critical fiction about the facilitation of professional and practice development plans in primary care. *Journal of Interprofessional Care*, **16** (4), 349–58.

Heard, S.R., Schiller, G., Aitken, M., Fergie, C. & McCready, H.L. (2001) Continuous quality improvement: educating towards a culture of clinical governance. *Quality in Health Care*, **10** (Suppl 2), 70–78.

Knight, P. (2001) Complexity and curriculum: a process approach to curriculum-making. *Teaching in Higher Education*, **6** (3), 370–81.

Magrab, P.R., Evans, P. & Hurrell, P. (1997) Integrated services for children and youth at risk: an international study of multidisciplinary training. *Journal of Interprofessional Care*, **11** (1), 99–108.

Pittilo, R.M. & Ross, F. (1998) Policies for interprofessional education: current trends in the UK. *Education for Health*, **11** (3), 285–95.

Reeves S. (2005) Developing and delivering practice-based interprofessional education: successes and challenges. Unpublished Ph.D. Thesis, City University, London.

5 The Curriculum

Developing an interprofessional education initiative needs to be well thought through and organised. It is a collaborative effort by the course development team to choose and build an appropriate curriculum and to disseminate their work during and following its completion. They need to be vigilant about the process of collaboration between the development team, members of which will have experiences of different professional backgrounds and institutional cultures.

Introduction

Next, we turn our attention to what the curriculum development team needs to do during their meetings and the tasks for individuals from that team. These, of course, are most often done between meetings. All this work ultimately results in a curriculum that will lead to effective interprofessional learning. Again, we realise that for some small initiatives, for example a single team training session, some of what we suggest will be irrelevant or over complicated. But interprofessional education always involves practitioners from more than one profession, so the development team will have at least two members. Our comments on developing a curriculum that effectively meets the learning needs of members of different professions and enables them to work better together are likely to help even the smallest initiative in some way.

It will not surprise you to read in this chapter not only about the items that will need to appear on the development team's agenda but also some of the ways to keep the team going as they work their way through that agenda. Bear with us if some of what we say seems familiar. Much of what you read about the planning team in the previous chapter also applies to the team that takes the curriculum development work forward towards approval (if that is needed) and ready for delivery to its students.

You will already have in mind some of the ways to make the most effective use of staff time and expertise. Remember that this especially applies to senior staff who will champion your work when resources and accreditation demand attention. Ask yourself who needs to be involved in the development process, when are they needed and how will they be kept up to date with your progress. The team may need to issue very brief management bulletins at key stages: who will take responsibility for this?

In Chapter four we suggested that not all the meetings need to be face to face, and that IT can provide an ideal communication tool when time is at a premium or geographical separateness of the collaborating organisations limits travel. Whatever the arrangements are, developing, then maintaining, team spirit and cohesion is important to the final outcome of the development process. That all starts before the development team have gathered for the first time, so if you have just skipped the previous chapter, consider going back. Jumping in without adequate preparation can be costly. In this chapter we will be building on the groundwork discussed in Chapter four and developing several of the issues we raised there.

First, though, let us look at the early development team meetings and some ways to make these a positive experience towards effective progress with the development of your interprofessional curriculum.

What you are developing and how to proceed with the development

The first meeting of the development team will influence the tone for the work of its members. Making time for each member to introduce her or himself and to confirm understandings of the task in hand and individuals' potential contributions may sound obvious items on the agenda. But in the rush to get going with the work that must be completed before the interprofessional education can be delivered, introductions and clarification are often neglected. The results can mean people feeling undervalued and confused, and working at cross-purposes with one another. While time given to sharing understandings and seeking clarification can feel as if the group is not making much headway with the 'real' work of developing the interprofessional education, the groundwork usually pays dividends, especially if you are planning a long or complex experience.

A formal way of approaching the work of planning an interprofessional course is to take an action-research approach, as reported by Stone *et al.* (2004). Two questions guided the development of their ethics course for students from seven health care professions. One focused on what should be included in the course (the content) and the other on what delivery design (or teaching and learning process) best suited the course content selected. You will recall that in the section on curriculum in Chapter three we discussed the relative importance of content and process in interprofessional education. This might be a good time to review these key concepts.

To answer the content and process questions, Stone and her colleagues tested the design for their course against their original criteria for content and process. One recommendation to emerge from the analysis of how the interprofessional education development team worked was the value of a systematic and deliberate approach to integrating new experiences into health care curricula. More examples of good practice in education planning and development can be found in the further reading list at the end of the chapter.

If the action-research approach feels too elaborate or too prescribed for your context, a simpler way to develop the interprofessional education, giving due attention to content and process, would use an agenda spanning several meetings, with items such as those that follow. These should not only be viewed sequentially, most need to be progressed and reviewed in parallel with one another. It should feel like a spiral of development that revisits key areas repeatedly, each time at a slightly more advanced stage. Our suggested key agenda items are listed as follows.

(1) Agreement over the planning process – sharing the conceptual model (or possibly a choice of models) for the development process discussed at the groundwork stage. This need not be elaborate, but if you are keen to use formal project planning tools we suggest you look back to Chapter four and our hints on these.

(2) Key personnel for the development team – a review of who has agreed to serve on the team and the identification of any gaps (professional, organisational, expertise), consideration of co-options keeping in mind the need for the team size to be a manageable and resource-effective. An ideal size is more than five and, according to Belbin (1981), not more than ten, as this creates a team that is too large for effective decision making. For interprofessional education planning and development, larger teams are often inevitable if all stakeholders are to be represented. If this is the case it is as well to be aware that group size may be the reason why your initiative is not as successful as you had hoped. We do not plan to repeat our comments on how teams work in this chapter, so you might like to take another look at what we say about this in Chapter four.

(3) Agreement on whether finding out about similar developments elsewhere will be of benefit and who is to be responsible for this.

(4) Consensus and clarity about the interprofessional learning experience under development, including the incorporation of interactive and adult learning methods and learning outcomes appropriate to interprofessional education.

(5) Clarification of funding arrangements and accountability.

(6) Course documents, for example background reading packs, discussion triggers, workbooks, assessment materials and other learning resources; and applications for academic accreditation or continuing professional development credit, transcripts of achievement or certificates of attendance, and so on: the why, what, how much and who of writing these.

(7) Recruitment and training of facilitators, tutors or mentors to deliver the interprofessional education.

(8) The process of gaining professional and academic accreditation, including, where appropriate, continuing professional development credit.

(9) Agreement about the approach to evaluating the initiative. This might include assessment of students, auditing changes in practice settings, and a formative or summative evaluation of the initiative of the type discussed in Section III.

(10) Considering how you will keep all the stakeholders informed about the team's work, for example by copying the minutes to them or alerting them to reports of key meetings posted on your project's website.

This is a rather general, and certainly not an exhaustive, list. Establishing one that is tailored to your particular context and desired development will be of much more use to you. The real danger is approaching course planning in a 'haphazard' manner (Stone *et al.* 2004 p. 61). If you and your team are unclear about the route you have taken towards your aim of effective interprofessional education, then it is much more likely that participants (learners and tutors) and anyone involved in accreditation might find some aspects obscure.

Later on in this chapter you will find a commentary on choosing curriculum content and processes and a guide to documenting the interprofessional education you are developing. The first and second items in our indicative agenda have already been discussed in the opening sections of the chapter. We look at learning methods and assessment of learning in the next chapter. Accreditation, staff development and evaluation get detailed attention later: for now we just want to prompt your thinking on these three issues.

- Your choice of curriculum, and especially the content and process aspects, may depend on whether you will seek accreditation for the interprofessional education you are planning; and the level of accreditation. Clearly there is a tangible difference in seeking accreditation that confers a licence to practice or a degree on students who successfully complete your interprofessional education, and seeking continued professional development credits for a short course or practice development initiative. If it feels that it will be too much effort to apply for continued professional development credit for a short initiative, or some interprofessional practice development, it is worth noting that the availability of these credits may attract funding and status, creating a positive impact on recruitment. Continued professional development credit also properly recognises the commitment of participants.

- Staff development and course evaluation share the need for early planning. All too often they take second place to the major work of curriculum planning until far too late in the planning process. Neglecting staff development when planning interprofessional education may mean that too few staff are sufficiently skilled and confident to teach or facilitate interprofessionally. For anything other than the smallest initiatives it is likely that you will need to recruit tutors and facilitators from outside the development team. Doing this early, keeping potential staff informed about the progress of the new programme and simultaneously arranging some staff development opportunities will be a key influence on the effectiveness of the programme. There is much more detail about this in Chapter seven. For now the message is to see it as a key part of course development, not a bolt-on extra.

- The need for early plans about how you will gather evidence about the effectiveness of your course is equally important. Poor questionnaires asking about how the participants found the 'day' or 'week' are often those that were put together at the last moment, or they have been plagiarised from another, possibly very different, course. This type of 'happy sheet' is exasperating for participants and does not yield well focused information for course developers. In Section III we discuss the evaluation of interprofessional education in some detail. Our belief is that robust evaluation design and sound measurement tools should be integral to the overall design and delivery of the interprofessional education. In this part of the book, where the emphasis is on programme development, we would encourage you not to forget evaluation nor postpone its planning.

But, to reiterate, our primary focus in this chapter is on the curriculum and everything we say from now on comes with a caveat about size.

Small is beautiful

One aspect of curriculum development that especially applies to interprofessional education and training is the undoubted value of starting small. In other words, think of your development as the pilot stage of a longer and more sustained project. You are, after all, aiming for effectiveness, and as we discussed in Chapter two, this means taking into account the need for positive outcomes, at an acceptable cost and without unacceptable side effects. Achieving an acceptable balance between these three elements usually takes time and openness to making minor changes, backed by evidence, in successive courses. In other words, reaching a state of effectiveness that is acceptable to all the stakeholders in Figure 2.2 is an evolutionary and iterative process.

So why start small? You may need to assemble a set of reasons that are specific to your course to convince managers and funding organisations of the value of piloting interprofessional education. Doing this does not mean that your initiative will remain small: only that this is the better way to start. This principle can be difficult to adhere to in the face of contractual issues and the demands made by education and service managers to deliver interprofessional education and training that meets current policy initiatives, and does so right now or, at least, tomorrow. There have been some notable exceptions to the small is beautiful rule, including the New Generation Project in the south of England (Box 5.1).

> **Box 5.1**   Interprofessional education in eleven health care professional
> programmes: the New Generation Project.
>
> The New Generation Project focused on the development and implementation
> of an integrated interprofessional education programme for all health profes-
> sional students studying at the University of Southampton and University of
> Portsmouth. The project aimed to provide students with opportunities to learn
> together during their pre-qualification education, to understand more clearly
> the contribution that different professions make to patient care and develop
> insight into the roles played by each profession. The interprofessional pro-
> gramme has been embedded in 11 separate professional programmes: audi-
> ology, medicine, midwifery, nursing, occupational therapy, pharmacy,
> physiotherapy, podiatry, diagnostic radiography, therapeutic radiography
> and social work. Each participating profession amended its curriculum to
> accommodate a number of short[1] interprofessional learning experiences,
> many in practice settings, and to provide well-timed preparation for the
> interprofessional education within the uni-professional part of the overall
> curriculum. It is important to note that the New Generation Project was
> made possible by substantial pump-priming funds from Government and a
> lengthy planning period. Formative and summative evaluation was embed-
> ded in the initiative. For further information and the latest news about this
> work see http://www.mhbs.soton.ac.uk/newgeneration

We are suggesting here that starting with a manageable and bounded initiative
may be more likely to be effective and practical. Your pilot course is like the acorn
from which the big oak tree can grow. As in nature, education benefits from
nurturing. Such attention is much more likely to lead to embedded, mature
interprofessional education and to the goal of effectiveness.

The interprofessional curriculum

There are a number of ways in which the activities associated with learning are
packaged in a cohesive way. These are referred to as the curriculum. Some of
these ways are substantial frameworks; others are based more on an ideology,
that is, on a system of values and beliefs, about the type of education that
underpins the design of the learning experience. The traditional and established
view of the curriculum arose within school-based education for children. It was
largely coherent and progressive, and excluded the views of the learners during

---

[1] This is the sense in which we see the 'small is beautiful' theme appearing even within this ambitious
and successful project. Short blocks of time are dedicated to interprofessional education and the
majority of each curriculum remains uni-professional.

the process of design and development. Classic curriculum models are either product (outcomes) orientated, led by objectives set for the learner; or process-driven led by hopes for certain types of student learning, including self-directed, experimentation and discovery-learning.

Concepts of the curriculum in adult education evolved out of this, for example Knowles' andragogical approach (Knowles *et al.*, 1998). This recognises the need to involve the learner in designing the educational initiative, planning their learning outcomes and assessing their learning. The teacher's role is to establish the learning climate, to support rather than teach and to acknowledge the learner's life-centred experience and their readiness to learn. This approach was used by Lia-Hoagberg *et al.* (1997) to underpin the development of their seminar-based interprofessional course designed to enhance teamwork knowledge for nurses, social workers, nutritionists and medical assistants. The authors noted that they undertook a needs assessment exercise before delivering the course, to allow these professionals to identify which topics were of relevance to their work.

Kolb's (1984) learning cycle is another model that links well with interprofessional learning. It places the emphasis on learning from and through experience and on reflecting upon such experiences. Freeth & Nicol (1998) outline how Kolb's work was used in an interprofessional initiative aimed at improving the clinical and communication skills of final-year medical students and newly qualified nurses, where the participants were given opportunities to discuss patient scenarios drawn from their clinical practice.

There are many more curriculum models and perspectives on curriculum design (underpinned by varying views on learning). In the further reading section you will find suggestions for texts that provide overviews of learning, curriculum design and evaluation. Many of the items recommended at the end of Chapter four are also relevant to this chapter.

The adoption of a particular curriculum approach should take into account the context in which it is to be used. Sometimes a combination of approaches is most appropriate. For example, it is possible to adopt a spiral curriculum, where topics are revisited and students build on what they have already learnt as those topics become more complex, alongside other approaches within the same curriculum (Bruner, 1977). Such a curriculum acts as a robust framework for progressively more difficult learning outcomes. It can accommodate the integration of a profession-specific core curriculum, the introduction of novel and individualised teaching and learning tools, like problem-based learning, and the inclusion of student choice in some subject areas (Davis & Harden, 2003). Another adaptation of the spiral curriculum can be found in the way interprofessional education has been woven into the ten professional undergraduate programmes offered at the University of the West of England (Barrett *et al.*, 2003). In this example the interprofessional element continues throughout the programme, with substantive interprofessional modules in each of the three years, interprofessional learning outcomes in uni-professional modules and supervised interprofessional practice. Finally, since interprofessional education frequently takes place in the work setting, it may be appropriate to use a work-based learning curriculum. Billet

(1996) provides a useful discussion on the nature of learning in the workplace, with its emphasis on active learning rather than teaching, and participation in communities of practice. This may be the most appropriate approach for your course to take if the aim is to enable practitioners to learn how work better together (see also Barr *et al.*, 2005).

Choosing a curriculum approach

One early decision for the development team is which curriculum approach they will take. Agreement about this means that course development can focus on issues of relevance in relation to key aspects of the selected curriculum. The preceding discussion should help you with this choice but do remember that our list of approaches is not exhaustive. There are alternatives that focus less on one of those generalised approaches and more on a theoretical rationale for the course you are planning. An example of this can be found in Box 5.2.

The evaluation of the initiative described in Box 5.2 led to conclusions about its efficacy and evidence that certain changes were needed. This example of using theory (in this case systems and group processes) to guide curriculum development shows that knowing why you develop the curriculum in a certain way leads to clarity about its components and enables post-evaluation, and therefore evidence-informed changes to be made.

Having a clear idea about the type of curriculum with which you are working will enable you to write and speak with confidence about the course to, for example, an approval panel or funding bodies. It will equip you with the means to explain the reasoning behind your planned course, giving rational explanations for the mode of delivery, duration, teaching style, assessment method, and so on, if your preparation and planning have proceeded well, with the added confidence that all those involved in the development of the course will offer a similar explanation.

Choosing the curriculum can be demanding when working interprofessionally. The sort of challenges that may arise during development team meetings relate to the unique aspects of each profession's philosophy, knowledge, skills and regulation, the need in interprofessional education for vigilance about language and culture, and the importance of recognising the different experiences that each professional brings. And for courses leading to academic and professional awards there is a potential conflict between the achievement of learning outcomes that support professional autonomy and those that focus on collaborative working.

You might like to brainstorm within your team about the reasons why professions develop their individuality and the sources of conflicts that often beset interprofessional education and collaborative practice. This can then lead into a discussion about how this might be addressed during the interprofessional education. The aim is for the development team to understand the roots of professional specialisation and professional conflict and ways of overcoming this. A realistic curriculum is more likely to emerge if this is the case, with tutors able to translate the written curriculum into the taught curriculum much more effectively.

Box 5.2   IPE for clinical improvement: a curriculum based on teamworking theory.

This Canadian study, reported by Irvine Doran *et al.* (2002), evaluated the impact of interprofessional training in continuous quality improvement methods for 25 hospital teams (= 150 staff) from a metropolitan area of Toronto. The educational initiative was guided by theoretical work on systems and group processes. It was designed to assist with the development of team norms. The aim of this was to promote effective interdisciplinary [sic] team-work, continuous improvement of patient care processes and planning of group performance strategies, and help participants to focus on mutual responsibilities in improving patient care. More theory was drawn upon to engage the teams in their quality improvement work, by reading literature that suggested using a structured framework for improvement initiatives and the value of making selected limited changes for which the impact can be evaluated.

The evaluation of the initiative was equally well planned, incorporating a waiting list control group, sound sampling rationale, and carefully designed and theoretically based instrumentation. Ethical approval was obtained for the study. The evaluation tested four hypotheses at the level of the teams; these were based on the belief that improvements in knowledge, team inter-actions, problem-solving abilities and patient outcomes should follow from the initiative. The first two of these were classified as immediate, the third as intermediate and the fourth achievable within four to six months.

The findings were reported, with attention to the study limitations, and included the observation that teams with physician participants were more likely to make changes in practice. From this the authors concluded that group composition is important in interprofessional teamwork. They also argue that changes in knowledge and team interaction do not necessarily improve team problem solving; suggesting that the content and approach of the interprofessional education may need greater emphasis on improving teamwork. The evaluation offered a contribution to understanding about the interprofessional nature of quality improvement initiatives in health care and drew out implications for management.

Such a curriculum will, of course, have, in part or whole, learning outcomes that relate to having the attitude, skills and knowledge to overcome boundaries and create transparent borders between staff from diverse practice settings; and to improve collaborative practice. These outcomes will shape the content of the curriculum (often also called the syllabus) and the teaching process. Table 5.1 suggests what sort of attitudes, skills and knowledge are needed for collaboration. The elements of this table will need to be adapted to the unique nature of your interprofessional education initiative but do use it to start thinking at an early stage in planning curriculum content and process.

Table 5.1 Attitudes, skills and knowledge for collaboration: a basis for interprofessional learning outcomes.

Pre-qualification	Post-qualification
Attitudes	**Attitudes**
Appreciate the value of interprofessional collaboration	Readiness to exchange viewpoints and information
Acknowledge other professionals' views and ideas	Willingness to share or relinquish responsibility
Knowledge	**Knowledge**
Understand the roles of other professionals and begin to identify how each professional role interrelates	Understand how professional roles interrelate
	Understand national and local contexts facilitating or inhibiting collaboration
Recognise the range of skills and knowledge of other professionals	Understand a variety of strategies for improving collaboration and the nature of underpinning logic models for change
Skills	**Skills**
Communicate with learners from other professions	Collaborate and negotiate effectively with other professionals and agencies
Identify situations in care where collaboration is helpful or essential	Identify situations in own working context where collaboration needs development; and act accordingly
	Select and adapt strategies for improving collaboration that are responsive to the specific care context

The learning outcomes are more likely to be achieved if you focus on ensuring that the participants have a positive experience of interprofessional education. Similarly, it is important to avoid setting people up to fail or to be distressed, which could turn them off collaborative practice. As with teaching and learning within and across different cultural settings, there is an advantage of sharing with students how the content of a curriculum will be delivered. In other words, students will benefit from knowing about the planned teaching processes and how you anticipate they will achieve the learning outcomes of the course. Learners new to interprofessional education may be meeting different teaching styles. They may differ in their experiences of syllabus delivery. For some, a series of lecturers, with handouts and tutorials may be the common pattern. Computer-aided learning, role-play, a problem- or enquiry-based approach, workshops and seminars may be more or less familiar to all or any of the students.

If you are planning a clinical or service-based interprofessional learning experience it is valuable to find out how teaching in service settings is usually delivered for the course participants. Teaching styles vary considerably across professional boundaries. Whatever you choose, we strongly recommend that the participants are made aware of this and are forewarned about the impact it may have on their ability to learn. New ways of learning usually take some getting used to. They take learners out of their comfort zone and can feel threatening.

Two other important influences on your choice of a curriculum are the need to link interprofessional education with the realities of practice for all the participants and to take account of the overall educational context of the inter-professional course you are planning. This later issue is much more significant in pre-registration programmes when, for example, an interprofessional module may be one among many uni-professional modules in each year or phase of an award-bearing programme. The case study in Box 1.2 is an example of this. Planning for an interprofessional module must include consideration of different ways the students' clinical experience is organised and the varying lengths of programme blocks (modules, placements, rotations, terms, semesters, etc.) for their respective profession.

You also need to take account of the priorities each learner will attach to any particular part of a long programme of study. When interprofessional learning outcomes coincide or conflict with other learning outcomes those that lose out are likely to be the ones thought of as lower status, those that are the least personally relevant or appealing to each learner, where the experience or assessment is most easily repeated later and learning outcomes are not assessed. The task of the interprofessional curriculum development team is to recognise the conflicting demands on learners and seek to avoid unnecessary clashes that might predict-ably divert attention from the interprofessional learning. The development team will also seek to strengthen the status and attractiveness of the interprofessional education by paying attention to learners' needs and the hidden curriculum.

Do try to anticipate how to deal with all of this if it has the potential to be a weak point in the interprofessional part of a longer programme of study. Allow time for the development team to explain to each other the ways in which their particular professional education programmes are organised and why. Try to explore arrangements that might mediate against a particular professional group of learners opting out of their team learning situation, which, of course, they might not do in body but might very well do in mind and spirit. One way of doing this is to ensure that your course optimises the strengths of different learning milieu and integrates learning within any classroom setting with that of the workplace or clinical skills laboratories.

Documenting the interprofessional course

Finally in this chapter we discuss briefly some key points about putting what you are doing on paper. Before starting to write ask yourself the following questions:

(1)   Why do you need to produce papers and documents about the course?

Answers to this may include:

    (a)   For scrutiny by appropriate academic, professional and regulatory bodies
    (b)   As recruitment material for prospective participants and their managers

    (c) To allow students selecting option modules to make an informed deci-
        sion about their choice

    (d) To form the basis of the students' handbook for the course

    (e) The course is innovative and worthwhile to share with colleagues in
        similar situations

(2) Who you are writing for?

Whatever your answer to this question, and there may be more than one, it is
essential to know your target audience for course documentation. This may be:

    (a) The learners who will take the course

    (b) Education managers within a funding body or higher education

    (c) Peer professional practitioners working on behalf of professional and
        regulatory bodies to accredit the course

    (d) Your colleagues and those who will teach and/or mentor students who
        take the course

(3) How much do you need to write and in what style should the course
    documents be written?

One way to find out how much to write and the preferred style is by looking at
previous examples of course documentation. What you need to remember with an
interprofessional course is that the different professional and regulatory bodies
and higher education institutions involved may well have differing requirements
of length, detail and layout. This is where the planning team will need to make
some decisions. Do you produce a happy medium with the risk that this will suit
no one perfectly? Do you produce documents tailored to each participating
profession? Finding out what others have done in similar circumstances can
prevent a lot of unnecessary writing. Do not be afraid to negotiate with committees and organisations that require documents from your team. Interprofessional
education is boundary-crossing work and the recipients of your documents may
well be prepared to engage with the spirit of collaboration and to some extent
vary their normal procedures and formats.

(4) Who will be responsible for writing these papers and documents?

This is a question that only the development team can answer. Don't forget that
this work can be resource intensive and the funding needs to be able to follow the
staff who have the time and experience to do this work. For a short course, or an
interprofessional quality improvement initiative, one person may offer to
write the planning meeting notes and take responsibility for converting these to
a set of course documents. Some of this can be done by administrative staff, but it
is worth remembering that the final responsibility for accuracy lies with the
course organisers and facilitators. For a long course, the writing is most usually
shared, with a senior member of staff acting as a coordinator for this work.
Again, some of the work might be given to administrative staff. They are often
very familiar with the requirements for this type of documentation and may be

much more at home with the technology available to produce clear and professional looking papers.

Posters, newsletter items, seminars, workshops and short reports at staff meetings are other opportunities to advertise the work of the planning and development teams. Perhaps someone in your team has a flare for leaflet design or writing press releases. It is worth investigating the strengths that lie within the development team so that the work of producing a wide range of documents and presentations for a wide range of audiences can be shared effectively.

Conclusion

Close attention to the type of interprofessional education curriculum you develop plays a large part in determining the outcome of the approval and delivery stages. Course development takes time. It shares many characteristics with the ways of learning new knowledge, skills and attitudes that it seeks to develop.

Key points

- Knowing the route you will take in developing your course and ensuring that the development team shares this knowledge is vital to the success of your development
- The choice of a curriculum needs to be made early in the process of developing interprofessional education
- The complex nature of interprofessional education means that the final product benefits from a pilot stage

Further reading

Boud, D. & Feletti, G. (1997) *The Challenge of Problem-based Learning*. 2nd edn. Kogan Page, London.

Kelly, A. (2004) The curriculum: theory and practice. 5th edn. Sage, London.

Light, G. & Cox, R. (2001) *Learning and Teaching in Higher Education: the Reflective Professional*. Chapter five: Designing: course and curriculum design. Paul Chapman, London.

Posner, G. (2003) *Analysing the Curriculum*. McGraw-Hill, Boston.

Scott, D. (2001) *Curriculum and Assessment (International Perspectives on Curriculum Studies)*. Ablex Publishing, London.

6 Learning and Assessment

The student's experience of learning and of ways in which that learning will be assessed need close attention in the development of interprofessional education initiatives. Understanding the key elements of interactive learning can help the development team to design a curriculum that maximises effective interprofessional learning.

Introduction

The work of the planning and development teams is aimed at effective learning for the interprofessional education participants. Previously, we discussed the groundwork needed for course development and the key factors influencing the type of curriculum your interprofessional team adopts (p. 75). Whatever curriculum approach you choose, the way the syllabus or course content will be delivered is one of its central components.

It is sometimes taken as obvious that teaching will lead to learning, but that link can be tenuous. To make your teaching effective it helps to know something about how people learn and in interprofessional education and training, how groups of practitioners from different professions most effectively learn with, from and about each other. In this chapter we look at some of the features that enhance learning in adults and other influences on effective learning in interprofessional groups. We also take a brief look at some of the principles that underpin assessing learning.

In terms of the 3P model (Chapter three) we are concerned in this chapter with examining *presage* to inform the design of the educational *process* that will meet your learning outcomes *(product)*. We will not arrive at a template for interprofessional education and its assessment because presage factors and desired products are unique to your context. We will be able to highlight common types of presage and to discuss several aspects of process. The examples within the chapter will show some of the variety that emerges when these common themes are applied in ways that reflect local needs and resources.

Learning as an adult

One important aspect of interprofessional education development is acknowledgment of the principles and processes that operate during learning and change, with the adult learner in mind. There is less of a division between concepts that underpin adult learning and learning in children than used to be thought. However, adult learners tend to be less subject to an external locus of control; they like to feel self-directed. Adults will usually be motivated and ready to learn when they have identified, or have been shown, a problem or challenge that interests them personally. Adult learners (and children too) tend to prefer active and interactive learning. They will bring a rich history of prior learning and experience to the interprofessional education and will want to feel that the facilitators and other participants value this. Adult learners also bring levels of self esteem, self-efficacy, and professional and personal identity that reflect their prior experiences. Some will approach interprofessional education very confidently, while others will be more tentative. Furthermore, adult learners bring baggage, such as unhelpful stereotypes, friction from the workplace, apprehension rooted in earlier unsatisfactory experiences, and hidden agendas relating to power.

A concise overview of some key texts on adult learning and their contribution to this subject can be found in Stagnaro-Green (2004), and other useful work is listed in the further reading at the end of the chapter. Here, we draw out a little of what we have said about adult learners in relation to developing and delivering interprofessional education.

Interprofessional education and adult learning

One priority is to develop interprofessional education around issues that the participants have previously identified; or around issues selected by the development team that are expected to be perceived as relevant to participants' learning needs. Typical challenges that become the focus of interprofessional learning include the coordination of multi-professional input to care for particular client groups (see Boxes 1.2 and 1.3) or at points of transition between care providers. Other foci might be quality improvement initiatives (see Boxes 1.4 and 1.6), or the evolution of roles and responsibilities within the multi-professional team (see Box 6.1).

Now might be a good time to look back at the spectrum of interprofessional education we discussed in Chapter one (see Figure 1.2). Your curriculum development team will need to examine its chosen topic and discuss whether it is planning an interprofessional learning experience that foregrounds improving interprofessional collaboration in the widest sense, using the course content as a vehicle for learning (an experience towards the right of the spectrum). On the other hand, the curriculum development team may be aiming to develop knowledge, skills, attitudes and workplace practices in relation to the chosen topic *and* add some value by doing this interprofessionally (an experience towards the left of the spectrum). Then again, the development team's aims might be more evenly split between developing interprofessional collaboration and developing practice for a particular context. We are not advocating a particular location on the spectrum as the most desirable. Rather, we are encouraging clarity of thinking during the development process. This way members of the development team are more likely to be striving for much the same end.

Another priority is to develop interprofessional education that promotes active and interactive learning; and values participants' prior experience. This precludes didactic teaching as a delivery approach. Instead interprofessional education employs small group learning techniques such as: workshop presentations with discussion; reviews of client case materials (real materials or a fictitious case created by experienced practitioners to draw out specific learning points); problem- or enquiry-based learning; simulation (varying from simple role-play to very sophisticated scenarios in real or lifelike settings); action-learning sets; development projects in practice settings or the wider community; intranet or Internet mounted discussion groups; and so on.

Effective interprofessional education requires high quality interaction, which in turn requires the opportunity for participants to listen, reflect, speak and be heard. Small groups working in small comfortable rooms would be ideal, but interprofessional education has to be delivered in a wide variety of settings. If you are catering for large numbers of participants in the most difficult environment of a very large tiered lecture theatre with fixed seats, they could first work in interprofessional pairs. Pairs can then become fours by working with those directly in front or behind. Large groups in large rooms with movable furniture are easier. Interprofessional subgroups can form around tables or flip charts while the facilitator(s) move from group to group. For very large cohorts it may be worthwhile using (and therefore paying extra for) a venue suitable for the number of students involved and the teaching and learning methods that an interprofessional curriculum demands. This was the approach taken by the University of the West of England, UK (Barrett *et al*, 2003, see Chapter five p. 74), who used a local conference centre to accommodate the large cohort of students enrolled on pre-registration interprofessional modules. This has the advantage of sufficient rooms for the many small groups for their formal work, and communal social areas for that important informal or serendipitous interprofessional interaction. Interprofessional education in practice settings also needs to be interactive. Box 6.3 shows the range of potential activities for interprofessional groups of students that can contribute to students learning with, from and about each other, staff and service users.

Valuing the prior experience of participants is partly a matter of prior planning and research, and partly an attitudinal matter when the interprofessional education is delivered. For the development group there is work to be done to anticipate who the participants will be, what their prior professional and interprofessional education curricula have addressed, which approaches to teaching and learning they are used to, whether they have identified learning needs that they hope the interprofessional education will address, and so on. In the opening chapter of this book we make the point that interprofessional education should not be seen as a one-off initiative. In other words, participating in just one interprofessional course, for example during their pre-registration degree programme, is unlikely to be all that is needed for practitioners to work collaboratively throughout their careers. In different settings, in the diverse roles they may have and at different times in their working lives practitioners may have learning needs that can be met by participating in education that is based on learning with, from and about their colleagues. The interprofessional learning cohort on your course may have vary-ing experiences of interprofessional education. This diversity may be in the quantity or the number of interprofessional events they have participated in and in their perceptions of the quality or effectiveness of this way of learning.

Learning about the potential participants in this way helps the development team to design an interprofessional learning experience that starts at the right level, neither undervaluing nor overestimating participants' prior knowledge and experience. It enables the development team to anticipate whether participants, or certain subgroups, will be unfamiliar with some of the planned approaches to learning and therefore might need additional support. This knowledge will feed into the timetabling, preparation of learning materials and staff development for facilitators, tutors, mentors and other learning support staff (Chapter seven). For example, it may be a good idea to include a discussion early in the course that alerts the participants to the potential discomfort they may feel, at first, with any new ways of learning, for example, those who have not participated in problem-based learning before. This will identify whether support is needed for anyone.

When the development phase research into participants' prior experience shows that they might well be predicted to find it hard to work together, or have difficulties engaging with certain approaches to learning, or that they have very different levels or types of prior experience, this would signal a need to consider addressing the areas of potential difficulty directly within the content of the interprofessional education. Participants may need to talk about their different ways of working, their differing views of what is important and the different ways in which they make decisions. It would also be advisable for the develop-ment group to seek out experienced and highly skilled facilitators to deliver the interprofessional education.

Ensuring relevance to participants' perceived learning needs, valuing what they already know and do, and promoting active and interactive learning are important aspects of developing and delivering effective interprofessional educa-tion. Happily, they are factors that are normally within the control of the educa-tion development and delivery teams. At the beginning of this section we also mentioned adult learners' preferred internal locus of control. This can be more difficult for the development team. Learners are not always going to be partici-pating in interprofessional education through choice. For some contexts certain courses are mandatory to help ensure safe and competent practice. At pre-qualification level it is increasingly common for interprofessional elements to be core components rather than optional experiences. Participation in interprofes-sional education at post-qualification level may be driven by peer or managerial pressure. Staff who develop and deliver interprofessional education should be aware that they might have reluctant learners. We mention this only because teaching an interprofessional group of participants with even just one person who arrives with a rather negative mindset can be a challenge.

We will say more about learner resistance later in the chapter. First, we discuss interactive teaching and learning, and keeping with the overall focus of the book we specifically look at what influences effectiveness.

Interactive learning

Where the aim is interprofessional learning, in other words learning with, from and about each other, it naturally follows that participants are dependent upon each other for at least some of their learning. This does not mean that individually they do not have responsibility for their personal and professional development. Rather, it is the very nature of interprofessional education, to a much greater extent than with other types of learning about professional practice, that the learning emerges from dialogue, discussion and debate within the group. The desired interactive learning may be achieved in a number of different ways as Table 6.1 shows. Each places different demands on tutors, facilitators, supervisors and mentors. Staff development to enhance their skills may be necessary (see Chapter seven).

Each approach also makes different demands on participants. The development team will need to reflect on these demands in relation to participants' prior experience and the time and support they will have. Attempting an approach that is unrealistic in the time available, or one that requires very high levels of support because it is completely alien to participants, may not be the best way forward. Learners like being stretched a little and put under a certain amount of pressure, but they do not like to face a high risk of failure. Your interprofessional education will be most effective if it is neither too easy nor too difficult. To judge this correctly the interprofessional education team will have to do its background research well to establish the interests, skills and experience of the anticipated participants. In addition, staff delivering the course will need to respond flexibly to any mismatch between the planning and reality as it unfolds.

We have already stressed that high quality interaction is important. In the group learning situation learner motivation, group balance, informal learning and learner resistance all have an impact upon the quality of interaction and collaboration, and through this on the achievement of interprofessional learning. We take a brief look at each of these key attributes.

Table 6.1 Types of interactive learning (modified from Barr, 1996).

Type of learning	Examples
(1) Exchange-based	Debates, seminar or workshop discussions, case and problem-solving study sessions
(2) Observation-based	Work shadowing, joint client/patient consultations (see, for example, Box 6.3)
(3) Action-based	Collaborative enquiry, problem-based learning, joint research, quality improvement initiatives, practice or community development projects, work-related practice placements for students (see, for example, Boxes 1.5 and 6.2)
(4) Simulation-based	Role-play, experiential group work, the use of clinical skills centres (see, for example, Box 6.4) and integrating drama groups within teaching sessions

Learner motivation

Many things affect learner motivation. Perceptions of the relevance and status of the course, whether participation is voluntary, the mode of delivery and teaching approaches are but a few.

The aim of interprofessional education is to improve collaborative practice (and thereby the quality of care). We have already said that in order to motivate participants to learn collaboratively, interprofessional education should be relevant to the participants' current practice (for post-qualification learners), or have perceived relevance their future practice (for pre-qualification learners and post-qualification learners seeking changed roles). The essential point about this attribute is that, as Thomas (1995, p. 212) argued, there needs to be 'fidelity between educational programmes and the real world'.

With this argument in mind, it is unsurprising to find that the majority of interprofessional education initiatives employ experiential learning approaches and are based wholly or partly in practice settings (more detail about the types and prevalence of interprofessional education can be found in our companion volume *Effective Interprofessional Education: Argument, Assumption and Evidence*, Barr *et al.*, 2005). Post-qualification learners may remain largely within their normal workplaces, or visit contrasting workplaces. Box 6.1 describes post-qualification interprofessional education developed through a partnership between a university tutor and frontline care staff, and delivered close to practitioners' clinical areas.

Pre-qualification learners may undertake placements in hospitals (for example Box 6.2) or in the community (see Boxes 1.5 and 6.3) or a simulated clinical environment (see Box 6.4). Even interprofessional education that is wholly classroom based tends to incorporate elements of simulated practice, for example role-play. Other aids to ensuring relevance include: pre-course information to identify participants' perceived learning needs and prior experience; timetabling activities within the interprofessional education that invite the sharing of experience, and activities that promote links between the interprofessional education and

---

Box 6.1   Post-qualification interprofessional education.

Carr *et al.* (2003) described an interprofessional education initiative where a university tutor worked with health care professionals in their clinical area to facilitate the development and delivery of an interprofessional education initiative designed to enhance the management of pain. A series of four study half-days were offered to staff at the hospital. In total, 72 members of staff from medicine, nursing, occupational therapy, physiotherapy and pharmacy attended one or more of these interprofessional sessions. Data collected by post-course questionnaires showed that participants valued participating in the sessions and sharing different professional perspectives on pain management. They felt they had gained helpful knowledge and insights.

Box 6.2 Interprofessional education in an acute clinical placement.

Guest *et al.* (2002) described an interprofessional placement in a paediatric ward within a large teaching hospital in the UK. The placement was developed for 90 senior nursing students and 90 junior medical students. It aimed to enhance students' understanding of one another's roles and responsibilities and to nurture mutual respect for each other's professional contribution to paediatric care. During the placement senior nursing students 'buddied' junior medical students. This allowed the students opportunities to gain insight into the realities of delivering care to patients on a paediatric ward. A qualified member of staff provided overall clinical supervision. The students' ward-based interprofessional learning experiences were subsequently discussed and reflected upon in seminar discussions. Questionnaires distributed to the students at the end of their placement revealed that all participants valued their interprofessional learning experiences on the ward. They also felt that there were improvements in their knowledge of one another and their clinical skills.

Box 6.3 Interprofessional education in a Canadian community placement.

Van der Horst *et al.* (1995) described the development and delivery of an early interprofessional community placement for pre-qualification students from a number of professional groups including medicine, nursing, occupational therapy, physiotherapy and social work. The aim of the placement was to enhance student understanding of interprofessional teamwork and improve their knowledge of the needs of users of community health services. Working in small interprofessional teams, students undertook a range of activities, such as observations of community interprofessional health teams, interviews with local community experts, interviews with the users of community health services, to gather information on teamwork and community-related issues. Students also attended seminars where their information was shared and discussed with their tutors and peers. Data gathered at the end of the placement revealed that the students enjoyed their interprofessional experiences. In addition, students felt that their knowledge of interprofessional and community issues was improved as a result of their participation in the placement.

---

participants' daily practice. For example, the use of drama groups to enact the realties of practice (including the perspective of the service user) can be a very powerful tool to initiate debate and discussion.

The perceived status and reputation of an interprofessional education experience can influence learner motivation. Attaining high status adds value and kudos to educational experience, which in turn makes it more attractive to

---

Box 6.4　Interprofessional education in a simulated environment.

Ker *et al.* (2003) described the use of a simulated ward environment for second-year medical and nursing students in Scotland. The ward was created in a clinical skills centre and based around simulated patients who displayed the symptoms of a variety of common medical conditions. After a briefing about the patients, students were allocated to interprofessional teams and were asked to take responsibility for the ward for a shift. At the end of their shift, the students prepared a joint report, which was presented to their tutors in the form of a ward handover. Student teams then received feedback on their performance by the tutors. Student questionnaires and observations of the student teams working together were collected. Findings from the evaluation revealed that students enjoyed working together in the simulated ward. It was felt that the ward provided a sufficiently realistic environment to help them learn about the demands of interprofessional collaboration when attempting to organise and deliver medical care to patients.

---

learners; helping to stimulate and sustain their motivation to engage in collaborative learning. This especially applies to post-qualification learners who generally have more choice over their education than pre-qualification students. There are a number of mechanisms for attaining a high status. You might be able to harness the support of high profile champions, particularly if they contribute to a session within the interprofessional education. The availability of valued learning materials, perhaps provided through the support of an external sponsor or through an arrangement with a commercial publisher will also add value. High quality tutors and accreditation for the interprofessional education (so that on successful completion it can contribute towards an academic award or the fulfilment of continuing professional development requirements) also signal value and kudos. We look more closely at accreditation in Chapter eight.

Low status problems have been noted for pre-qualification interprofessional education. Here, those elements which aim to enhance collaboration can be perceived as having lower importance for students in relation to their primary focus on learning their own professional roles, knowledge and skills. Dienst and Byl (1981) provided an early but insightful example of the nature of this problem. In their evaluation of a community placement for pre-registration medical, pharmacy, nursing, physiotherapy and dental students, these authors found that students regarded the development of their own profession-specific skills as far more important than developing their teamwork skills. Consequently, most students spent little time participating in teambuilding sessions. They preferred to spend time enhancing the clinical skills associated with their own profession.

Learner motivation may also be low when interprofessional education is attached to low status elements within a curriculum rather than high status elements; or low status practice environments rather than high status practice environments. For example, Pryce & Reeves (1997) found that first-year students who undertook an interprofessional community-based placement viewed community care as a low status area for learning when compared to the prospect of learning in acute care settings. Your curriculum development team will know (or will be able to find out) the relative status of the curriculum elements or practice areas that they might choose as sites for embedding interprofessional learning. The team should not necessarily choose to avoid low status elements and practice areas; the interprofessional education may be a very good way to improve their standing. Nevertheless, the team should be alert to the possible connection between status and motivation.

Another facet of status and motivation is assessment. If only some areas are assessed in a curriculum with many elements, the subliminal message to learners (the hidden curriculum) is that the non-assessed elements are not as important as the assessed elements. This may not be true. It could be that the non-assessed elements are rather difficult to assess and that this challenge is yet to be overcome. Interprofessional education often falls in this category. We will return to assessment later in the chapter. Reeves (2000) offered some insight into the link between resistance, motivation and awarding credit. His evaluation of a community-based interprofessional placement for pre-qualification nursing, medical and dental students, found that the nursing students, unlike their medical and dental peers, did not receive any educational credit for completing the interprofessional course. This resulted in reduced motivation and increased resistance among the nursing students.

As we mentioned earlier, voluntarism is another of the attributes that can have an important effect on learner motivation. This especially applies in pre-qualification education, where learners may have little choice about when or how they participate in interprofessional education. Lary *et al.* (1997) argued that choice should be given to students whether or not they embark on a programme that includes interprofessional education, but, at least in the UK, such choice is denied as a matter of Government policy. All pre-qualification health professions' programmes of study must now contain some interprofessional education. When there is no choice the perceived relevance and status become more important. These, in turn, depend on the mode of delivery, approaches to teaching and providing students with information about the aims and benefits of the interprofessional elements.

For post-qualification learners the issue of voluntarism has a different set of implications. Qualified practitioners usually select what type of continuing professional development they wish to undertake. However, there are examples of interprofessional education, implemented by clinical managers to overcome poor clinical practice, where staff are expected to participate. For example, in their evaluation of the implementation of an interprofessional quality improvement initiative to improve the care of patients with depression, Rubenstein *et al.* (2002) described how lead clinicians from two managed care primary care clinics in the USA worked with evaluators to develop and roll out an initiative with interprofessional elements. Encouragingly, they found that medical, nursing, social work and other staff in both clinics supported their managers and interacted well together during their interprofessional learning sessions about the implementation of the initiative. And, as the initiative became more embedded in the practice of their clinic, staff continued to collaborate well together.

On rare occasions, it has been found that staff can resist management-driven interprofessional education. For example, Hunter & Love (1996) described an evaluation of an interprofessional quality initiative designed to reduce inpatient violence in a USA forensic hospital. Staff initially resisted a number of the suggested modifications to practice that emerged from the quality improvement process changes, for example management attempts to have voting rights for the patient representative in the quality improvement team. However, the authors went on to note that after further negotiation with the staff group, explaining the need to have a 'consumer perspective', the initiative was ultimately accepted.

It is worth doing a *voluntarism check* on the education or training initiative you are developing. Remember, the more diverse the professions represented and the greater number of agencies represented the more likely it is that some may be there just because they have been sent.

Group balance

Another aspect of developing effective interactive learning is the need for group balance. Three facets promote good interprofessional interaction: group stability, group leadership and group profile. By profile we mean the professional mix, the numbers from each profession and overall group size.

In an interprofessional group made up from largely one profession, interaction may be inhibited, especially if the larger professional group can dominate. This effect can be accentuated or dampened by the relative status of the majority group. Nevertheless, many development teams have to face the challenges of imbalances in the size of the learner groups. For example, the nature of health care means that there will always be far more pre-qualification nursing students than occupational therapy students. Conversely, for a post-qualification practice development initiative in primary care there may be far more doctors than practice nurses.

The development team needs to be aware of the impact of uneven numbers and status differentials on the interaction of the learning group and to discuss potential ways to overcome the challenges these imbalances present. With skilful facilitation, minority groups, and particularly those with relatively low status, can be encouraged to contribute their experience and will feel that their perspectives are valued. Members of minority groups may be called upon (or feel compelled) to contribute proportionately more than members of the majority group in order that their profession's voice is equally heard. Drawing attention to the stressful nature of this for individuals can help to ensure that work is more fairly distributed.

Small group learning will be more effective if the participants work together in a coordinated way. This applies to their collaborative effort on the tasks they are asked to do and also to any contributions they may make to plenary sessions. This type of work usually benefits from some organisation and someone taking the lead. Within any group leaders usually emerge naturally, as do members willing to take the other important roles in a team. We discussed team roles in Chapter four and it might be worth looking back at that section with the learning group in mind. Within the interprofessional learning context participants often come from a practice background with a strong tradition of leadership from particular professionals. Gender, age and seniority all influence expectations about leadership. Interprofessional education is an arena in which assumptions about leadership, and any associated tensions, can be examined and challenged. Longer interprofessional learning opportunities offer scope to try out rotating leadership.

The balance of the group is also affected by group size. Small groups are undoubtedly preferable. Gill and Ling (1995, p. 187) put the case for this well by arguing that:

> 'Interactive processes require that students are able to talk with each other without having to raise their voices, are able to establish eye contact, feel sufficiently confident both to express their opinions and to explore uncertainties in front of others from different professional backgrounds. These conditions, however, are seriously compromised by large groups which preclude such intimacies.'

The investment demanded by small interprofessional groups may be challenging to acquire, especially in an educational climate that requires costs to be contained. Nevertheless, you should be aware of the impact of group size upon the effectiveness of the education initiative you are planning. Hughes & Lucas (1997) recommended learning groups of around eight to ten members. They reported poor quality interaction when their groups comprised more than ten members.

The final facet of group balance is the need to maintain stable group membership. This can be especially difficult in post-qualification interprofessional education. Heavy workloads can mean that stability is interrupted, as practitioners are not able to attend all the sessions of a course or practice development initiative. Another disruption is when the bleep calls one or more participants out of a session. If this is likely during your initiative then it would be worthwhile spending some time looking at ways to minimise these problems. Can other people hold the bleeps and screen calls for a short while? The timing of the sessions can make a significant difference, although there will never be a time that is good for everyone. Combining group work with the availability of lunch may make a key difference.

Another method of maintaining group stability is to offer interprofessional education on a residential basis, where clinicians can be taught without the daily pressures of their workload interrupting their learning (see Box 6.5). However, this option is relatively expensive and requires a greater time commitment from the participants and their work colleagues.

In contrast, for learners undertaking full-time pre-qualification education, the pressures on group stability should be less severe. But there can be attrition and absenteeism. Students may be absent due to illness or changes in personal circumstances. There can also be significant absenteeism if the interprofessional education has low status (perhaps signalled by lack of assessment), is inconveniently located or timed, is delivered in an uninspiring or anxiety-provoking manner, or coincides with important assessments in other course elements.

Informal learning

A further factor is the informal learning, which takes place before or after the formal learning activities are undertaken. Such learning can provide students and practitioners with valuable opportunities to share and debate aspects of their formal learning in a more relaxed fashion. You might like to think about how to build informal opportunities for learning into the programme you are planning, for example making arrangements for participants on a short course to have lunch together and ensuring that time is available for students to socialise. LaSala *et al.* (1997, p. 295), for example, pointed out the importance of the local cafeteria as a useful setting for 'informal sharing of impressions and experiences' among pre-qualification students. In addition, they noted how students 'car-pooled' and used the travelling time to and from the university to work together on their group project.

Box 6.5　Residential interprofessional education.

Long (1996) provided an insight into the effects of delivering a three-day interprofessional residential course for members of two primary care teams consisting of general practitioners, practice nurses, practice managers, district nurses and health visitors. The aim of the course was to provide an opportunity for teambuilding and to provide a catalyst for enhancing collaboration. It was decided that the course should be offered to both teams on a residential basis to ensure that members could focus on their interprofessional learning without the distraction of work pressures. Time away from work was negotiated with colleagues, who deferred their attendance to another time. Interviews with the course participants revealed that they valued the course for providing them with time to understand each other's professional roles and responsibilities. It was also felt that the course allowed them to start communicating in a more systematic manner.

Learner resistance

As outlined above, resistance is another factor that needs to be taken into account when developing an interprofessional course. It is worthwhile the development team discussing whether resistance is anticipated; considering who or which groups may be resistant, how resistance might be displayed and the reasons why resistance to interprofessional education arises. The following list of reasons, collated from a number of different courses, may help you begin this discussion.

For pre-qualification, learner's resistance can arise because:

- Collaborative learning is not perceived to be as important as profession-specific learning, and it interrupts profession-specific learning
- The need to learn about teambuilding is an additional burden, and teamworking skills are considered marginal to other practice skills
- Interprofessional education is potentially threatening to self-identity and self-esteem.

Learner resistance tends to be different in post-qualification interprofessional education. It is often more open and obvious; with palpable suspicion of interprofessional workshops in clinical settings. This is unsurprising. Interprofessional education is generally introduced into these environments in anticipation that it will change and enhance present practice. It can be perceived as a possible indicator that current practice is inadequate. Where the interprofessional education has been initiated by managers and specifically designed to develop and/or change ways of working this can be perceived as a criticism of professional behaviour and a challenge to professional autonomy.

Gelmon *et al.* (2000) offered a typology of learner resistance, reproduced in Table 6.2. If you have had experience of learner resistance, take a few moments to identify whether it appears in Table 6.2. Can you relate this to the course you are

Table 6.2 A typology of resistance applied to interprofessional education (Gelmon *et al.*, 2000, p. 134).

Stages	Examples of resistance
(1) Acceptance	Cooperation
	Passive resignation
(2) Indifference	Apathy
	Doing only what is being ordered
(3) Passive resistance	Regressive behaviours
	Protests
	Working to rule
(4) Active resistance	Doing as little as possible
	Committing errors
	'Spoilage'

presently working on? Can you find ways to prevent the participants on the new course from being or becoming resistant?

Strategies to overcome resistance include recognising the unique contribution each practitioner makes to care and reinforcing the value of this within the collaborative approach to work. It is also useful to provide more resistant learners with reminders about how to change their practice and offering further educational input. For example, Nolte *et al.* (1998) described how they overcame staff resistance to a quality assurance initiative designed to enhance the management of medication for cancer patients by offering follow-up interprofessional education sessions to staff. McCoy *et al.* (1997) outlined a similar approach overcoming resistance in an initiative designed to improve the quality of patient documentation. Finally, the explicit commitment of both professional leaders and managers is fundamental in overcoming practitioner resistance.

Assessment

Formal assessment of changes in knowledge, skills and attitudes during or following interprofessional education is undeveloped. This status probably relates to the relatively new nature of learning with, from and about each other, as a distinctive aspect of professional education; the complexity of measuring interprofessional collaborative competencies; and the challenges of uneven availability of interprofessional learning opportunities. During course development you and your team will need to debate the concept of assessing interprofessionally and work towards a consensus about implementing interprofessional assessment. For some courses this means sophisticated assessment procedures capable of satisfying academic, professional and regulatory bodies.

Assessment should be capable of not only differentiating between successful and not so successful learners but also enabling learning and improvement. This is most usually achieved via a formative feedback system such as written comments or sensitive tutor-participant discussions, which can add considerably to staff workloads. The development team needs to take account of the resources that feedback will demand.

When we talk of assessment enabling learning and improvement this is because we are conscious that assessment has a large and not necessarily positive effect on learning. There are several features of assessment that can distort the learning experience, including the timing, frequency, format and the sort of knowledge or behaviour that it implicitly rewards. For example, interprofessional education is largely concerned with effective collaboration but the most familiar and well-developed systems of assessment actively discourage collaboration – we usually call that plagiarism. What we are describing is a lack of constructive alignment between the assessment and the learning outcomes. The challenge is to develop assessments that are well aligned with the desired learning outcomes (Biggs,

2003). Ideally, the assessment of learning should be an integral part of the learning process. Many aspects of interprofessional education require sophisticated assessment: employing methods that are relatively underdeveloped within and beyond interprofessional education, for example the assessment of an individual contribution to the product of a learning team.

In some instances formal assessment of participants' learning during interprofessional education will not be necessary. For example, an initiative designed to improve the quality of service offered by a health care team should be judged by changes in quality indicators for the service. We would not be particularly interested in isolating and measuring individual learning. Nevertheless, some relatively informal formative assessment might be motivating or provide additional coaching and therefore assist the realisation of the principal aim of improving the quality of the service.

Self assessment or peer assessment within an interprofessional group or team could communicate to the learner how they are doing without the threat that the tutor or organisation 'will know what I don't know'. However, self and peer assessments can be far more brutal than most tutor assessments.

Any course that confers academic or professional credit and an award is likely to need more formal assessment procedures and to include ways of summarising the student's learning (summative assessment). One way to approach the design of the assessment for a course is to ask the following questions.

- Why is it necessary to assess the participants' learning?
- What aspects of learning from the interprofessional experience do we wish to assess?
- What assessment tools are appropriate for the learning outcomes?
- Are these tools acceptable in terms of validity, reliability and practicality?
- Is there authenticity within the content of the assessment items?
- Is there constructive alignment between the learning outcomes, the learning process and the assessment processes?

Given the difficulty of assessing interprofessional education outlined above, only a few initiatives include some form of assessment. These include:

- Team handover, where learners provide verbal feedback on their interprofessional learning experiences to their tutors (Ker *et al.*, 2003, see Box 6.4 above)
- Individual written assignments that describe and evaluate the process of working together in an interprofessional team (Bezzina *et al.*, 1998)
- Poster presentations, whereby learners collate salient aspects of their interprofessional experiences on a jointly designed poster that they present to tutors (for example Reeves, 2000)
- Multidisciplinary team treatment care plans, whereby learners jointly develop a collaborative approach to the delivery of patient/client care (Brown & Adkins, 1989).

If you want to look further into assessment in higher education, Brown *et al.* (1997) explained many of the basic concepts and provide details across the width of assessment methods presently used in adult education.

Conclusion

Our discussion has focused on two keys aspects of any curriculum: approaches to teaching and learning, and the assessment of that learning. More than anything else these aspects of the student experience influence the outcomes of the education. Learning experiences that involve participants from different professional backgrounds and the complex demands of learning interprofessionally have the potential to generate fear of failure. This may turn participants off collaborative practice. An awareness of this by the curriculum development team and a willingness to give adequate time and careful thought to the participants' experience of learning and assessment plays a large part in the achievement of effective learning.

Key points

- Interprofessional learning is influenced by the motivation of the participant and any resistance they may have to this type of education.
- The make-up of the interprofessional learning group plays a key role in the effectiveness of the education.
- The outcome of interprofessional education is strongly influenced by the ways in which the knowledge, attitudes and skills needed for collaborative practice are learnt.
- Assessment of interprofessional education is complex and presently under-developed.

Further reading

Biggs, J. (2003) *Teaching for Quality Learning at University.* 2nd edn. SRHE & Open University Press, Buckingham.

Boud, D. & Feletti, G. (1998) *The Challenge of Problem-based Learning.* 2nd edn. Routledge Farmer, London.

Eraut, M. (1994) *Developing Professional Knowledge and Competence.* Falmer Press, London.

Gibbs, G. (1992) *Improving the Quality of Student Learning.* Technical and Educational Services Ltd, Bristol.

Jarvis, P., Holford, J. & Griffin, C. (2003) *The Theory and Practice of Learning.* Routledge Falmer, London.

Knowles, M., Holton, E., & Swanson, R. (1998) *The Adult Learner: the Definitive Classics on Adult Education and Training (Managing Cultural Differences)*. Gulf Publishing, Houston.

Light, G. & Cox, R. (2001) *Learning and Teaching in Higher Education: the Reflective Professional*. Paul Chapman, London.

Moon, J. (2000) *Reflection in Learning and Professional Development: Theory and Practice*. Routledge Falmer, London.

Shumway, J. M. & Harden, R. M. (2003) BEME Guide 25: the assessment of learning outcomes for the competent and reflective physician. *Medical Teacher*, **25** (6), 569–84.

7 Staff Development

Initial preparation and continuing support of staff makes a vital contribution to the success of an interprofessional education initiative. Attention to staff development ensures that those delivering and supporting the curriculum have the appropriate knowledge, attitudes and skills to undertake their roles and responsibilities. The aim is to develop skilful facilitators, who adapt to participants' and colleagues' skills, experience and interests; and understand the issues of power and hierarchy inherent within the everyday practice of working interprofessionally. Whilst facilitators are the lynchpin of interprofessional education, other groups may also benefit from development opportunities.

Introduction

The preparation and continuing development of staff who support and facilitate interprofessional education is essential if the initiative is to achieve its aims. Normally, these people will also be supporting and facilitating uni-professional education, so they will have well-established, relevant skills and knowledge. However, interprofessional education is different from uni-professional education, sometimes in quite subtle ways, which creates a need for its own staff development. This is all too easily overlooked.

In this chapter we address the nature of initial preparation and continuing support for staff working at professional interchanges. We briefly address the needs of support staff and champions, but our main focus will be on the group that might be thought of as 'teachers': tutors, facilitators, mentors and supervisors to name but a few titles and roles. You will find references to examples of what is currently available to help people learn the craft of teaching interprofessionally. However, while instruction and observation are very helpful, development ultimately occurs through *doing* and *reflecting* on action and reaction.

Teachers, tutors, facilitators, mentors and supervisors

The vibrant and demanding task of facilitating interprofessional learning requires skills in a unique and often challenging blend. We would argue that this calls for staff development and support for teaching interprofessionally as an inbuilt part of the development of interprofessional education. In this way it can add value to the work of the development team as the curriculum they have planned is implemented effectively. Thinking ahead like this militates against staff development being seen as an optional extra, added on at the end, or, in the worst case, a rescue package when the teaching and learning is in trouble. But first we need to establish who the interprofessional educator is likely to be and why staff development plays such a key role in the success of their practice and effective learning for their students.

People with many years of experience in facilitating uni-professional learning may recreate the way they were taught or experiment with different approaches when asked to facilitate interprofessional education. Professions and disciplines tend to have characteristic ways of doing things, so the facilitators are likely to have internalised norms, preferences and expectations from the professional group to which they belong or normally teach. Their established educational role may be closely aligned with profession-specific knowledge or skills. Their expertise may lie within just one of the spheres of activity that the planned interprofessional education will draw upon. Their experience may be rooted in a curriculum that demands interactive teaching and learning, giving them insight and practice in facilitating group learning. Others may have taught on shared learning courses or met mixed student groups on clinical placements. Yet others may only have worked in an expert–apprentice relationship with students of their own profession. Then these educators choose to embrace interprofessional education, or find themselves allocated to this task.

In an ideal world interprofessional educators will:

- Have experience in group facilitation.
- Have experience of team teaching or co-facilitation, preferably with colleagues from other professions or disciplines.
- Have experienced a professional development pathway that has given them a strong commitment to, and realistic views about, interprofessional learning and working.
- Be skilled at foregrounding aspects of collaboration while valuing the distinctive experience and expertise of each of the participating professions.
- Be attuned to the dynamics of interprofessional learning and competent to help groups through conflict and disaffection.
- Have had experience in the context of practice that the interprofessional education is aligned with and have developed some expertise in the competencies needed for skilled and safe practice in the setting.
- Be skilled in optimising learning opportunities that arise from everyday practice and in helping learners make connections between theory and practice, and between different areas of practice.
- Be accustomed to helping learners to overcome miscommunication that arises from different professions' underlying perspectives and use of language.
- Be comfortable with the learning and teaching methods and technologies that are part of your initiative: possibly including facilitating action-learning sets or

problem-based learning, supporting and appropriately blending learning, making effective use of simulation, using video feedback, encouraging attention to process as well as content, and so on.

- Be familiar with constructively aligned assessment, able to contribute to the development and delivery of innovative assessments and skilled in providing well-targeted and sensitive feedback.

Of course there will not be very many of these fully formed interprofessional educators available. Your colleagues may possess an uneven and partial mix of these qualities. Finding out what things they are good at, what they feel confident about, along with those things in which they need support and structured experience, is a good place for the development team to begin to identify staff development needs and possibilities. For example, needs might include interactive teaching and learning, facilitating learning that is not based on the facilitator's profession-specific expertise; understanding group dynamics; handling conflict and using it productively; working with reluctant learners, or using unfamiliar technologies.

The expertise to deliver staff development addressing these needs may well be available within the development group or from local experienced facilitators. Facilitator development might proceed well on a self-help and mutual exchange basis, or more formal workshops may be preferred. In a spirit of interprofessional collaboration, participating organisations may make their existing staff development opportunities available to staff from each of the participating organisations.

Exceptionally, you may need to allocate funds for external training. Provision of staff development in this area is diverse, embracing work-based learning, continuing professional development programmes and formal award-based programmes. For example, in the UK, CAIPE offers staff development workshops based on a great deal of experience across many different health and social care settings. Moseley (1997) described a short UK-based university-led interprofessional course that aimed to prepare tutors as effective interprofessional facilitators. The content focused on understanding different professions' roles and responsibilities, exploring issues of professionalism and their effect on interprofessional learning processes, and planning learning strategies that could be employed when facilitating an interprofessional group. Mhaolrúnaigh and Clifford (1998) described another UK-based university course designed to enhance the facilitation skills of nursing, midwifery and health visiting tutors, and Clay *et al.* (1999) described a USA-based university course for health care tutors designed to enhance their confidence and expertise in facilitating interprofessional groups.

Being an experienced and well respected facilitator or practice supervisor for one profession does not necessarily signal an unproblematic transition to interprofessional education. The transition may reveal insecurities and limitations that were masked in the other setting. This calls for sensitive development and ongoing support.

From time to time interprofessional education may be the first educator role undertaken by a practitioner. These facilitators will need staff development for the interprofessional aspects of their work and more general development and support for teaching and learning. Such support for teaching and learning roles may be available from one or more of the participating organisations. Professional development for teaching and learning is often offered to multi-professional groups and should be sufficiently interactive to constitute interprofessional education. This will give the novice educator first-hand experience of learning with, from and about members of other groups. A novice educator may also benefit from an experienced mentor, particularly one with experience of interprofessional education.

The development team will need to consider whether all types of interprofessional educators can share staff development activities or whether certain groups, for example practice supervisors and assessors, have very specific learning needs that are better addressed separately. Hook and Lawson-Porter (2003) provided an example of interprofessional staff development involving eight professionals assessed and accredited by a UK university. Participants, all with a health or social care qualification, were currently in practice and were prepared to have students on placement. The three-day course provided 24 hours contact time, with 75 hours directed study. Topics covered during the taught element included models of supervision, problem solving and conflict, and assessing competence. Evaluation of this ten credit undergraduate module identified the need for flexible delivery, the value of the interprofessional nature of the course and that the participants' practice with students had changed positively. Ongoing educational supervision for practice educators from the university was seen to be desirable.

Managers and champions

Effective interprofessional education needs institutional support at many levels. The 'front line' staff are likely to become very despondent if their efforts to work collaboratively are thwarted or unrecognised by colleagues and/or their organisation. Managers at all levels can help to ensure that the efforts of the curriculum development team blossom into valued and effective interprofessional education. For this to happen, the development team may need to inform a variety of management groups about the aims, advantages and support needs of the planned interprofessional education. Of course this is a two-way process, with the curriculum development team learning from the perspectives of those groups.

Anticipating the need to offer staff responsible for the strategic direction of teaching, learning and practice development in the participating organisations the opportunity to explore some fundamental issues about interprofessional education may be one vital step in ensuring the success of your initiative. For staff at very senior levels it is necessary to think creatively and integrate development opportunities with other events, for example as part of meetings they already attend. You may consider an invited speaker, someone with credibility, a reputation that will encourage full attendance and who has at least a chance of positively influencing tutors' and managers' thinking towards the goals that the development team is hoping to achieve.

Support staff and services

Interprofessional education crosses organisational and professional boundaries, but support services may be very much tied to working within their own institutions. Advertising the course, registration of participants, collection of fees and payment of staff, provision of learning materials, room bookings, timetabling, the processing and verification of assessments, IT support and library access are all aspects of interprofessional education that challenge support staff and services. This is because its boundary-crossing nature is not catered for in systems, procedures and service agreements. More importantly, it is often just not part of people's routine thinking. Informing support staff and services about the aims of the interprofessional education, where it fits with existing provision, and why it is necessary for it to be different from everything else they deal with, will enhance the important role they play in education provision. Once more the education should be two-way. You and your team will have to learn about existing systems and service contracts and the ways in which the planned interprofessional education will fit into these, or the initiative may run into difficulties.

Why is interprofessional teaching development necessary?

We have just made a strong case for staff development for all those involved in interprofessional education. In the next section we look in detail at some of the issues that give rise to these developmental needs. If you are planning an interprofessional staff development event think about the value of raising these issues with the participants. This means exploring areas that may feel uncomfortable and challenging to those involved. This can be mediated by small group discussions, ensuring that the group members set some ground rules such as confidentiality, giving each member a time to speak and listening attentively. The list of issues we have chosen is not exhaustive and there may be others that your students can think of that would benefit from similar sessions.

Scepticism

Some staff may be sceptical about a new interprofessional education initiative, especially since evidence for its effectiveness is only recently available and is not yet comprehensive (see Chapter two and also Barr *et al.*, 2005). These staff may hold rather negative views about interprofessional education and yet, in many circumstances, not have a choice about taking a role in the teaching or learning support teams. Their reality may be one where the introduction of interprofessional education has been done to meet policy imperatives. They may have had little or no influence about the curriculum that is now in place for their students.

Confidence and credibility

To work confidently interprofessional educators need to feel secure about that part of their knowledge base that will be drawn upon during the education, and sure of their ability to facilitate the learning of heterogeneous groups. We identified, in Chapter one, that heterogeneity (diversity) is part of the uniqueness of interprofessional education. Educators can feel vulnerable if they anticipate that their knowledge, values, assumptions and pedagogic skills will be challenged by learners' and colleagues' differing sets of prior knowledge, different expectations about the ways in which education should be conducted, and possibly different aspirations for outcomes arising from interprofessional education.

Of course, the diversity among participants also provides many learning opportunities and unusual constellations of expertise that can be used creatively to develop new insights and new approaches to challenges in the delivery of care. Nevertheless, drawing out insights and new approaches from the collective wisdom of a diverse group is a highly skilled task. It requires a range of strategies and constant 'reflection-in-action' (Schön, 1987) to select strategies wisely and flexibly in response to the dynamics and progress of the group. No wonder that some tutors and facilitators feel apprehensive about engaging with interprofessional education. Particularly so when their skills might, through the medium of interprofessional co-facilitation, be on display not only to the course participants but also to colleagues from neighbouring practice areas or academic departments. Confidence can be built through shared staff development that examines the intended learning outcomes for your initiative and explores ideas about useful approaches to facilitating learning and strategies for addressing any anticipated problems.

The facilitators will need to establish their credibility with the learners in relation to their knowledge of the focus of the interprofessional education and their ability to facilitate interactive learning. Facilitators who work mainly in universities may struggle to maintain credibility in professional practice. This may undermine their confidence or the learners' confidence in them; particularly practice-based, post-qualification learners or students with recent practice-placement experience. Staff development needs include ongoing contact with the practice contexts that the interprofessional education was developed to serve. On the other hand, highly respected practitioners may be inexperienced or under-confident facilitators who need supportive staff development. Your team may find that the contrasting staff development needs can be met through work shadowing, short role exchanges, workshops or briefings delivered by members of the curriculum development team, or from within the pool of facilitators, or co-mentorship (possibly combined with co-facilitation) between practice-based and university-based pairs of facilitators.

Staff development in interprofessional teaching is about awareness of the opportunities and frustrations within the target practice contexts. In other words, it also means knowing quite a lot about interprofessional and inter-agency collaboration in practice, teamwork and participative working.

Spotlighting personal professional knowledge

Course leaders and managers also need to be aware of how vulnerable facilitators may feel working with colleagues from other professional groups and the weight of the responsibility for effective learning of students from less familiar professional backgrounds. The professional baggage we all carry may have its downsides but it does give us an inbuilt confidence. Instinctively we know certain things about the sources of our own professional knowledge and its application. All practitioners have tacit (or hidden, unrecognised) knowledge of their professional practice. This is passed on, albeit less obviously, to the next generation of practitioners. It is not unusual for teachers or mentors with many years experience of uni-professional education to remain unaware of this. Unaware, that is, until they notice how different it can feel facilitating a team of health and social care learners where diverse ways of knowing surface and other languages are used to explain core concepts and practices.

Interprofessional teaching puts this difference between our own and others' professional knowledge in the spotlight. Used positively it can help us to understand the complexity of interprofessional learning. If teaching interprofessionally is a challenge, how much more so, then, is learning in this way. But it also has the potential to undermine our confidence in our teaching skills and can become a barrier to the development of a sound relationship between tutors and interprofessional learning groups.

Sharing responsibility to reduce risk

Often the initial success of an initiative depends largely on a handful of talented key enthusiasts, staff who are willing to dedicate their time, often outside the working week, to develop and nurture an initiative; staff whose energy, enthusiasm and experience help to make the interprofessional education highly successful. In extreme circumstances the interprofessional education may be planned and delivered by one person. This is a risky strategy. When enthusiasts move on there may be nobody well placed to ensure that the interprofessional education continues to be successful. This would be highly wasteful of the resources committed to development and the lessons learnt from the initial cycles of curriculum delivery and evaluation would be lost from the participating organisations. The curriculum development team (and as we said earlier, we think it should be an interprofessional team, however small, in preference to an individual) should attend to staff development that will safeguard the continuation of the interprofessional education initiative. High quality development work needs to be embedded and not left vulnerable to the loss of champions or partner organisations. This means early attention to the professional development of a pool of facilitators drawn from all the partner organisations.

Role models

As in so many other situations educators are role models for learners in inter-professional education. It is not difficult to see how facilitators and support staff collaborate among themselves and between groups. Their responses to learners will influence the strength of the collaboration between learners. This will apply across a range of behaviours, in the classroom, in practice settings and during social exchanges. It can happen consciously and unconsciously. Staff development can raise awareness of role modelling and its impact on learning.

Perkins and Tryssenaar (1994) pointed out that one useful approach to provide a good example of interprofessional role modelling is shared facilitation. This can model the behaviours the interprofessional education aims to develop by showing that facilitators trust one another and value each other's contributions. Of course, poor quality shared facilitation can undermine the aims of the interprofessional education and avoiding such problems can be a good focus for staff development.

Crow and Smith (2003) implemented co-teaching for post-qualification health professional students from diverse settings on an undergraduate degree in health and social studies. The learning environment created by this approach had two key features. First, there was a similarity between the attributes of interprofessional co-teaching and those that are important in interprofessional collaboration, namely, trust, respect for each other's views, openness and an awareness of the influence of personal professional discourses. Second, the dialogue between the two teaching staff created an active learning environment in which ideas were openly discussed, one hallmark of interprofessional education. The authors conclude that the dialectic between the co-facilitators acted as a powerful role model.

Teaching effective interprofessional education practice: the challenges

To reprise our introductory argument, effective interprofessional education demands that educators make good choices about how to teach an interprofessional group of learners and implement these choices effectively. Putting their decisions into practice, even with a confidence based on careful planning and personal preparation, can still be demanding. Many educators will know about the principles of adult learning and their experience in applying these will be invaluable for facilitating interprofessional learning. However, more than that is needed, including an insight into personal and professional attitudes, language and values, sensitivity to deeply held beliefs in our colleagues and a willingness to move forward differently.

Competencies for interprofessional teaching

It is possible to view the competencies needed for effective interprofessional teaching as a model with two interdependent aspects (see Box 7.1). On one side there is the need to be aware and realise the learning potential of interprofessional group dynamics. This is matched by the responsibility to provide opportunities for effective individual learning for each member of the group.

Acquisition of these competencies, and any additional ones that are specific in your context, will provide a solid foundation of staff development to support your interprofessional education.

Ways of organising teaching support for interprofessional learning

The above discussion will have given you some clues about some of the topics to include in a staff development course. One thing will have become clear during your reading of this chapter, namely, that the skills of facilitation are essential, and without these the potential to positively affect collaboration will be diminished. The following sections take a brief look at some of these.

Facilitation strategies

To support collaborative learning facilitators need to pay attention to team formation and team maintenance.

Box 7.1   Competencies for interprofessional teaching.

- A commitment to interprofessional education and practice
- Credibility in relation to the particular focus of the interprofessional education to which the educator contributes
- Positive role modelling
- An in-depth understanding of interactive learning methods and confidence in their application
- A knowledge of group dynamics
- Confidence and flexibility to use professional differences creatively within groups
- Valuing diversity and unique contributions
- Balancing the needs of individuals and groups
- Inner conviction and good humour in the face of difficulties

---

Team formation

Specific strategies are available to aid the team formation process. For example, 'ice-breaker' and teambuilding activities, and exploring learners' initial expectations of interprofessional education to ensure any differences are discussed and resolved. Facilitators need to be ready to encounter interprofessional friction between learners. Problems can arise between learners, particularly in 'sensitive' areas such as misunderstanding other professional roles or perceived 'overlap' into another group's professional domain. When this happens, Thomas (1995) suggested that the facilitator should accept this 'confrontation' and should devote time to exploring and discussing the issues and their effect on collaborative learning within the group. We would argue that awareness of the nature of diversity between interprofessional education participants, initially sought out at the planning and development stages (Chapters four and five), and refined as the interprofessional education progresses, allows proactive use of the diversity in teaching and assessment strategies (Chapter six).

To overcome any initial anxieties and fears learners may have about working together with members of different professions, facilitators need to establish a learning environment which is supportive, relaxed and where everyone's input is equally valued (Cleghorn & Baker, 2000). Creating (at least temporary) 'equality' may be more important in post-qualification interprofessional education, where individuals come together to learn together from differing positions in organisational hierarchies. Funnell (1995, pp. 168–9) argued that:

> 'An important aspect of [the] initial planning may be the creation of learning groups of individuals who perceive themselves as equal, irrespective of their particular position in their own organisation. Such an arrangement has the potential for facilitating peer bonding and encouraging sharing.'

Equality among participants is an important facet of the 'contact hypothesis' that underpins a number of interprofessional education initiatives, including those for which the Interprofessional Attitudes Questionnaire was developed (see Box 11.3). (We discuss the contact hypothesis, and other theories that underpin the development of interprofessional education, in our companion volume Barr *et al.* (2005) and there is a short explanation in the glossary to this book.) Achieving equality among participants at the team formation stage may be a question of skilful allocation of individuals to subgroups. It might also be achieved by early discussion of the importance of everyone's contribution being valued and the need to temporarily set aside 'baggage' from the workplace, negative stereotypes, and current hierarchies.

Team maintenance

A number of strategies are available to maintain collaboration between learners and maximise opportunities for equality within interprofessional learning groups. These include rotating the position of group leader (Funnell, 1995) and offering more autonomy to groups during their learning, thus giving control of the learning initiatives to the group itself (Thomas, 1995). This enables the group learning processes to be seen as more closely resembling the self-direction, autonomy and interconnectedness of professional practice in service settings. Such an approach was adopted by Howkins & Allison (1997) in their interprofessional course for doctors, nurses and social workers. In their post-course evaluation it was found that participants enjoyed being given control over their own learning, with this being one of the 'most significant factors' in the success of the course (p. 229). However, some learning groups will need more 'hands-on' facilitation to help overcome, for example, pre-existing conflict, large power differentials, or inexperience with self-directed group learning.

Conclusion

This brief discussion has touched on several of the important issues related to staff development in interprofessional education. Your staff development programme needs to be tailored to your local context and to the aims of your particular interprofessional education initiative. We would suggest that you review our suggestions against the backdrop of the local context and aims early on in the development process, so that staff development needs can be allocated sufficient resources and developed for timely delivery. Ways to enhance interprofessional learning need to be explored by those who will have educator and support roles. A multifaceted staff development programme that draws from expertise within the partner organisations, often from within the curriculum development team, will smooth the path for delivering effective interprofessional education.

Key points

- Staff development for interprofessional education should be inclusive, embracing practice educators, university lecturers and those with administrative and managerial responsibilities.
- Interprofessional education creates a need for staff development that is shaped to the local context and the aims of a particular interprofessional initiative.
- Interprofessional teaching demands insight into personal and professional attitudes, language, and values, a sensitivity to deeply-held beliefs in our colleagues and a willingness to move forward differently.
- Staff development for interprofessional education aims to reduce any scepticism held about new ways of delivering professional education and enhance the confidence and credibility of staff involved in its delivery.

Further reading

Brockbank, A. & McGill, I. (1998) *Facilitating Reflective Learning in Higher Education.* SRHE and Open University Press, Buckingham.

Eby, M. (2000) Understanding professional development. pp. 48–69 In: *Critical Practice in Health and Social Care* (eds Brechin, A., Brown, H. & Eby, M.) Sage, London.

Edwards, H., Baume, D. & Webb, G. (eds) (2003) *Staff and Educational Development.* Kogan Page, London.

Jaques, D. (2000) *Learning in Groups: a Handbook for Improving Groupwork.* 3rd edn. Kogan Page, London.

Knowles, M., Holton, E. & Swanson, R. (1998) *The Adult Learner.* 5th edn. Gulf Publishing Company, Houston, Texas.

Light, G. & Cox, R. (2001) *Learning and Teaching in Higher Education: the Reflective Professional.* Paul Chapman, London.

McGill, I. & Beaty, L. (2001) *Action Learning: a Guide for Professional, Management and Educational Development.* Revised 2nd edn. Kogan Page, London.

Ramsden, P. (2003) *Learning to Teach in Higher Education.* 2nd edn. Routledge, London.

Salmon, G. (2004) *E-moderating: the Key to Teaching and Learning Online.* 2nd edn. Routledge, London.

Savin-Baden, M. (2003) *Facilitating Problem-based Learning: Illuminating Perspectives.* SRHE and Open University Press, Maidenhead.

Schön, D. (1987) *Educating the Reflective Practitioner: Toward a New Design for Teaching and Learning in the Professions.* Jossey-Bass, San Francisco.

8 Testing your Development

In this chapter we discuss ways to check the quality of planned interprofessional education. We encourage internal reflection on the curriculum, that is, self-assessment by the course development team, and also provide an insight into formal approval of the quality of curriculum development by universities and professional bodies.

Introduction

You will recall from Chapter two that two of the characteristics of educational effectiveness are positive outcomes without unacceptable side effects. Both of these are very general. In this chapter we look at their translation into specific criteria for high quality education for your particular interprofessional education course. We continue by outlining the features of the processes that universities and professional bodies use to assess, and thus to approve, professional education and, of interest to us, interprofessional education. In focusing on formal approval we have not lost sight of the fact that many interprofessional learning initiatives remain informal. For these the self-assessment process is the main quality mechanism.

Effectiveness, quality and approval: the ties that bind them

This book is all about achieving effectiveness in interprofessional education. Earlier chapters in this section aim to help you towards effectiveness during the development of a course. Here we encourage you to reflect upon the work that you have done and on the product of that work. Our goal is to give you a start as you consider:

- What constitutes effective interprofessional learning?
- What makes a sound and high quality interprofessional learning experience?
- What characterises effective interprofessional education?

We would also like you and your colleagues to be comfortable with the ideas and practice of self-assessment and external approval as a means to enhance the quality of the interprofessional education you have developed. In this respect we suggest that you work interactively with your product: to assess the potential for effectiveness of your course, to measure its quality and take a reflexive stance about the curriculum that you plan to deliver. We also hope that you will share your experience with others in similar situations and will be able to learn from the experience of others.

We discussed earlier how effective interprofessional education should have a positive effect on the learners and not produce any unacceptable side effects. It is more usual to evaluate those effects that can be measured in the short term, such as positive changes in knowledge and development and an enhancement of skills, than it is to assess whether there are any long-term and unacceptable side effects. This is always done in retrospect, looking back at the results of the initiative, at learning and its impact on practice. Here we look at what you can do in anticipation of the interprofessional education to give some assurances to the participants and other stakeholders that the course or event will be, at least, good enough and, hopefully, effective. We look at the nature of quality in interprofessional education and discuss what various stakeholders will look for in your curriculum (Chapter two p. 33–4) and preparatory staff development (Chapter seven) to provide sufficient confidence that they will get value for the resources and commitment they plan to invest. Later we provide a list of quality questions to guide the curriculum development team's self-assessment and preparation for the scrutiny of others.

Self-assessment and informal peer review

Testing your curriculum with a steering group (which may have been formed at the end of the initial planning stage, see Chapter four) is a useful aid to self-evaluation among the curriculum development team. Explaining plans, progress and the rationale for decisions to others is a good way to test your own understanding and the coherence of the development team's work. Gaps and inconsistencies become obvious. Colleagues with experience of the approval process may be available to offer their thoughts. Through discussion within the development team, between the development team and the steering group, or between the development team and a wider range of colleagues, the gaps and inconsistencies can be addressed.

Seeking the views of appropriate external examiners or consultants are two other ways of obtaining informal peer review of the worthiness of the curriculum your team has developed. Publications and relevant organisations, such as CAIPE, are ready sources of advice and expertise that can be used as you proceed through the process of assessing the quality of your planned interprofessional education. CAIPE has a development manager, who acts as a point of reference for help, and an accredited panel of consultants and trainers to advise at all stages of the development and accreditation process.

We will shortly discuss approval by professional, regulatory and academic bodies. Even if you do not plan to seek approval from one of these you can often access information about their quality questions, criteria and processes from their websites or print resources. This material can provide guidance for self-assessment.

Formal and informal scrutiny by resource providers

Any of the stakeholders whose perspectives are highlighted in Figure 2.2 might provide resources to support interprofessional education and they will engage in varying degrees of formal scrutiny of the product of their investment. For example, local budget managers and staffing coordinators may only require a convincing case to be presented (either verbally or as a short document) before they will exercise the discretion to support your initiative within their roles and available resources. The partner organisations are likely to require scrutiny by operational and strategic committees before new resources are secured or existing resources are redirected to support your interprofessional education. External resource providers are likely to scrutinise the curriculum, a business plan and the development team's risk assessment of factors affecting the delivery of the planned interprofessional education. In all cases effective interprofessional education has to be achieved at an acceptable financial and human cost.

Scrutiny from potential participants or their representatives

The interprofessional education participants (learners, facilitators and service users) dedicate time and effort, and possibly money and emotion. Where there is free choice, they will only choose to participate if their scrutiny of the opportunities offered gives reasonable hope of gains for individuals and groups. These gains may take the form of, for example, improved collaboration in the design and delivery of services, new knowledge and skills, insights into the perspectives and contributions of others, or simply an enjoyable experience. Where there is choice, market forces should help to enhance the quality of interprofessional education. Where there is no choice, or severely restricted choice, other quality mechanisms will be required to permit scrutiny and influence from participants. For example, reference groups of participants' representatives might be established. The curriculum development team would consult these at key stages in the development work. The reference groups might also contribute to the planning and execution of evaluation (Chapters nine and ten) when the planned interprofessional education becomes a reality. Another mechanism for securing ongoing scrutiny from representatives of interprofessional learners, facilitators and contributing service users is through direct appointment to the curriculum development team. Where this occurs these members of the group could be given a central role in monitoring the development team's self-reflection.

Scrutiny from professional, regulatory or academic bodies

Professional, regulatory or academic bodies that in any way endorse your professional education will be investing part of their reputation and credibility. Naturally, these organisations will require some assurances that your planned interprofessional education deserves their approval (which may also be called accreditation or validation). Normally they do this before the interprofessional education commences. Even if approval follows a pilot experience with the interprofessional education, the approval process is still highly likely to precede the availability of anything other than early formative evaluation (Chapters nine and ten). Therefore the scrutiny will normally focus on the aims, objectives and design of your interprofessional education, in addition to its content and resourcing. Approval processes may also consider the credibility and capability of the facilitation team, underpinning support for learning and teaching, assessment designs and systems, the track record of the partner organisations, market research and risk management strategies.

Approval processes most usually include an element of peer review. The professional and statutory bodies and higher education institutions call upon experienced and willing education and practice-based staff to undertake this on their behalf. Interprofessional education initiatives often need or wish to seek approval from more than one organisation and this often means more reviewers than for uni-professional awards or single subject degrees. Just as the names given to the approval process vary, the systems, procedures, timescales and documentation required by different approval bodies vary. This can be problematic when the same interprofessional course requires multiple approval. The curriculum development team will need to be aware of differences between the bodies so that the needs of each are met with as little conflict and duplication of effort as possible. We will return to this later.

Quality questions

One way of assessing the quality of your interprofessional education is through an interrogation of the curriculum you have designed. An honest look at the answers to a plain set of questions such as those (adapted from Barr, 2003) that we set out below, will give you a clear picture of whether what you plan to deliver has a sound rationale and is in tune with the principles of interprofessional education.

- Are the learning outcomes designed to promote knowledge, skills and attitudes appropriate for collaborative practice?
- If it is part of a wider educational experience how is interprofessional learning built into the whole?
- Is the interprofessional learning informed by a theoretical rationale?
- Are the teaching and learning methods within the curriculum shaped by current best practice in interprofessional education? A review of some the

material in Chapters six and seven will guide you towards answers to this question.

- Do the values of interprofessionalism permeate the entire curriculum?
- Are the learning methods interactive?
- Is there sufficient small-group learning?
- Will numbers from the participant professions be reasonably balanced? Where this cannot be so, what will be done to support minority groups?
- Were all the professions represented during curriculum development and will each contribute to the curriculum delivery?
- Are patients and carers involved in the planning of the course and will they participate in its delivery?
- Is the assessment of interprofessional learning compatible with the approaches to teaching and learning?
- How will the results of the assessment contribute towards the qualification awarded on successful completion of the course?
- What plans are there to evaluate the programme?
- How will the evaluation results be shared with the community of practitioners in interprofessional education?

Approval processes: pre-qualification

Methods for seeking approval of an educational course and the ways this is given depend on many things. Features of the interprofessional initiative, for example the type of course, who the participants will be, its intention and duration, or how the learning material is to be delivered, will all determine how approval is obtained. In almost every instance the process includes peer review and scrutiny of curriculum documents. Understanding the reasons why approval is important and, possibly essential, is key to a successful outcome. For example, in the UK all pre-qualification programmes that confer an academic and professional award on the successful student require approval by the appropriate academic, regulatory and professional bodies.

These different bodies confer approval for different reasons. For those most relevant to interprofessional education it is worth noting that:

- University validation takes place to ensure that courses comply with university regulations and that there is consistency across courses and between higher education awarding bodies
- Accreditation by professional or regulatory bodies confers the recognition that a course provides the competencies needed for professional practice

In other words, university validation focuses mostly on ensuring that the student is fit for the award, and the professional or regulatory bodies on whether the newly qualified practitioner is fit and safe for practice. It can be very challenging to meet the individual requirements of fitness for award and fitness for practice.

Seeking approval for interprofessional education within a pre-qualification curriculum will lead to scrutiny of the learning outcomes to which it contributes and the means of assessing these. There will also be concern about any learning outcomes from elsewhere in the wider curriculum that might be 'squeezed out' by the interprofessional learning objectives. Be ready to defend what the proposed interprofessional education will add to the wider curriculum, what steps have been taken to avoid overload, and the validity of any proposed assessment. For almost all initiatives it is the case that uni-professional curricula are remodelled or repurposed as interprofessional rather than being replaced by something entirely new. It is valuable to be able to show how this applies to your proposal.

As we stressed in Chapter seven, there should be as much harmony as possible between the aims of the interprofessional education and its assessment. This suggests newer and less conventional forms of assessment that allow students to demonstrate constructive collaboration or skills for collaborative practice. While traditional assessment methods, such as the essay question, are likely to be approved with little debate, the innovative assessments that you may create to achieve constructive alignment with interprofessional learning objectives are likely to generate rather more unease and debate. Imagination and persuasive ability are likely to be required, along with professional judgement about how much change and risk the approval panel is likely to tolerate. Innovative assessments need strategies for the fair treatment of students who do not complete the assessment satisfactorily, whether through absence or poor performance.

Approval processes: post-qualification

More and more professional and statutory bodies have mechanisms for the recognition of post-qualification, postgraduate studies and for shorter episodes of continued professional development. Interprofessional education needs to be part of the collection of continued professional development courses, events and activities that are accredited by the professional and registration bodies. Needless to say, across the multiple professions in the health and social care sectors there are multiple approaches to this. One professional or statutory body may lack interest in your interprofessional initiative, another will operate a postal approval system and another may demand extensive course documents and want to send a team to discuss the curriculum with you, perhaps even visiting participating practice areas. It might be possible to use one set of documents and meetings to satisfy the requirements of two or more approval bodies, but you may have to face the possibility of separate approval processes running in parallel for each relevant approval body. This will lead to (possibly hard-fought) decisions about which approval bodies are the most relevant. Agreed division of work among the curriculum development team and good communication between those engaged with separate strands of work will be essential.

The reality of the approval process

Approval processes are often stressful for the course development team. For most the outcome is successful and there is cause for celebration of a job well done. The process can take a long time and may involve a lot of bureaucracy. Staff see themselves and their work as under investigation and this can feel a lot worse than it is meant to be. Planning and preparation is the key to successful approval. Nowhere is this more necessary than for the complex and challenging validation events that are often associated with the academic and professional approval of interprofessional learning for two or more health and social care practitioners. Arrange pilot events, informal peer reviews of documents and ensure that your team all know and believe in the course being presented. Do try to seek support from senior faculty staff for the development team. These are the people best placed to offer the members of the approval panel assurances about the financial and other partnerships between education and service settings that will underpin the effective delivery of the planned interprofessional education. They are not necessarily required to be present during all of the approval meetings. Sometimes their role as the hosts at lunch, with the opportunity to meet and briefly talk to the approval panel members, is all that is needed.

Mostly, there is a pleasant and collegial atmosphere and the approval panel work with the clear intention of being helpful and positive. Occasionally the panel turns out to be a little adversarial in nature. Awareness of this possibility by the course development team is helpful. Do find out about the experiences of colleagues so that you have an idea about the working methods of panels from particular organisations. Be prepared for different approaches from individual members of the approval team. Representatives of different stakeholder groups may be trained very differently in their roles. These differences will apply to the way they will comment on the documentation about your course. Some will be much more concerned with the values that underpin your approaches to interprofessional education and the translation of these through the design of the curriculum. Others may focus on specific details, such as the assessment procedures or the student handbook.

The alternative role

You may be reading this book because you have been asked to participate in the approval of an interprofessional course as a representative of one of the bodies referred to above. This section is written for you and has a slightly different focus to the rest of the chapter. This does not mean that as a member of an approval panel you will work to different criteria of effectiveness from the staff who have developed the educational initiative. Such an arrangement would clearly be counterproductive and unethical. The list of quality questions we suggest above (p. 113) is likely to be just as useful to someone on an approval panel as it is to someone developing an interprofessional educational initiative. Approval processes are not there to 'catch people out' and should not be confrontational. Our assumption is that approval panel members aim to be helpful, supportive and willing to listen to the course team as they present the rationale and structure of their course.

Your responsibility as a panel member is to ensure that the approval process is another example of collaborative working. It is valuable to remember that knowledge of interprofessional education still varies within and across institutions and professions. Different practitioners have varied experiences of interprofessional education and in some professions it remains contested.

An understanding of what effective interprofessional education really means is rapidly evolving, but there remain gaps in knowledge about what works for different professional groups, and in what circumstances, highlighting the need for evaluation and dissemination (Chapters nine to thirteen). Interprofessional education is, at best, a developing pedagogy. In these circumstances it is wise to encourage creativity in course design and delivery, and diversity in the ways that interprofessional learning outcomes are achieved. The important thing is that the course development team can offer supported arguments for their choice of curriculum design and implementation.

Conclusion

Approval by at least one academic, professional or regulatory body may well be necessary for the interprofessional education initiative you are thinking of developing, or have already developed. Even if external approval is not needed, it is good practice to be reflective about the final curriculum design and to interrogate the curriculum in ways that can highlight whether or not it will achieve its intended aims. In this way, the answers to some questions about the quality of the initiative can give insight into whether it will have an effective outcome for the course participants.

Key points

- Successful accreditation is much more likely when the course development team are well prepared for the scrutiny of the interprofessional initiative.
- For short courses external peer review may not be required. Here the course development team will need to be reflective about their work and take time for self-assessment of the resulting curriculum.

- The course development team and the reviewers are working towards similar criteria of effectiveness and quality indicators.
- The approval process is much more effective if it takes place in an atmosphere of collegiality and when all involved have the common aim of ensuring that the outcome for the participants will be interprofessional learning.

Further reading

Biggs, J. (ed.) (2003) *Teaching for Quality Learning at University*. 2nd edn. Open University Press, Buckingham.

Brennan, J. & Shah, T. (2000) *Managing Quality in Higher Education, an International Perspective on Institutional Assessment and Change* (particularly Quality assessment in higher education: a conceptual model, pp. 9–18.). OECD, SRHE, Open University Press, Buckingham.

Quality Assurance Agency for Higher Education (2001) *Benchmarking Academic and Practitioner Standards in Health Care Subjects/Professions*. Quality Assurance Agency for Higher Education, Gloucester.

Quality Assurance Agency for Higher Education (2002) *Benchmarking Academic Standards in Medicine*. Quality Assurance Agency for Higher Education, Gloucester.

Quality Assurance Agency for Higher Education (2001) *Benchmarking Academic Standards in Social Policy and Administration and Social Work*. Quality Assurance Agency for Higher Education, Gloucester.

Smith, H., Armstrong, M. & Brown, S. (1999) *Benchmarking and Threshold Standards in Higher Education*. Kogan Page, London.

Stephenson, J. & Yorke, M. (eds) (1998) *Capability and Quality in Higher Education*. Kogan Page, London.

Section III
Evaluating the Effectiveness of Interprofessional Education

Introduction

Current emphasis on evidence-based practice within health and social care directs attention towards evidence for the effectiveness of interprofessional education. Such evidence is building up, but progress is slow, particularly in respect of the *processes* that underpin effective interprofessional education and its *longer term impacts*. In part this is because there are so many interrelated variables in any teaching and learning process, not just interprofessional education. Nevertheless, the evidence base is expanding and improving all the time. We say more about this in our companion volume Barr *et al.* (2005).

Sound evaluation of your interprofessional education developments will help you to establish the worth of your work and improve future development and delivery of interprofessional education. With a strong design, insightful analysis and appropriate dissemination, your evaluation could also make a welcome contribution to the growing knowledge base of the interprofessional education community. In the following chapters we take a detailed look at the evaluation of interprofessional education initiatives, but first, let us dwell for a moment on the word 'evaluation'.

Evaluation, research, audit, quality improvement

These terms, and perhaps others you can call to mind, are closely related and are sometimes used interchangeably. While distinct definitions for each could be provided, the important thing is that they each have connotations of understanding, judging and explaining something with a view to seeking improvement. Some terms sit more happily in certain environments than others. It is rarely necessary to be very concerned with the semantics of these different terms, but it is worth remembering that different terms mean different things to different people and this can impair communication. Working in the interprofessional education arena this frequently applies to the type of education being discussed, but associated activities, such as obtaining evidence for its effectiveness, are just as likely to benefit from terminological clarity.

Take a moment, now, to think about your reactions to different evaluation-related terms and the impact of decisions that might flow from these. The following example may help to focus your thoughts.

'Our clinical area is engaged in rapid quality improvement cycles, including interprofessional training, to address our service delivery improvement objectives. To evaluate our progress we are going to conduct an audit to look for improvements . . . We won't be doing research so we don't need research ethics committee approval and we are not looking at research methods books or training.'

- How do you react to the evaluation-related terms in this account?
- Do you think your colleagues from a range of professions would react similarly?
- Are research and evaluation really different things?
- Are the judgements sound in relation to the necessity of obtaining research ethics approval and the pertinence of the research methods literature?

For simplicity, in this book, we have settled upon the term 'evaluation' to describe the processes of systematic gathering and interpretation of evidence, from which judgements can be made and ways of promoting improvement recommended.

As with the discussion of curriculum and the work of a curriculum development team in Section II, at first glance it may appear that our focus is on larger-scale, multifaceted and longer-term evaluations, but first appearances may be deceptive. Whilst we do want to encourage multifaceted and longer-term evaluation of interprofessional education it does not have to be large-scale. Chapters nine to twelve initially highlight the important decisions in the process of planning an evaluation and then we discuss the essential aspects of the lived experience of evaluating. Their content is not overly technical or complicated. What we have to say nearly always scales down, remaining pertinent to single-handed evaluators working on small projects. Our focus is on well-planned evaluation appropriate to the local context.

9 Planning Sound Evaluations

Planning a sound evaluation is a multifaceted, iterative process that takes longer than most people recognise. Investing time and attention in preparation gives a firm foundation, helping to ensure a smooth running, well-targeted, efficient and useful evaluation. This chapter focuses on the range of evaluation designs that have the potential to answer questions about the effectiveness of interprofessional education, influences on your design of choice and the process of arriving at these fundamental decisions. This early work is then further shaped by external forces and agents as discussed in Chapter ten.

Introduction

The evaluation of interprofessional education involves the *systematic* examination of interprofessional learning opportunities and experiences, *permitting thoughtful judgements* of effectiveness and other aspects of value, and *promoting improvement*.

Promoting the improvements that stem from judgements about effectiveness and value are key aspects of professional practice in health and social care. While considering varying conceptions of effectiveness in Chapter two, we noted that ensuring appropriate evaluation of interprofessional education can be seen as a professional and ethical duty for those who commission, develop and deliver it. Appropriate evaluation that aims to meet the needs of stakeholders in the interprofessional education process (including those highlighted in Figure 2.2) can be achieved in many ways. You need to be able to make informed choices about evaluation designs, the allocation of appropriate personnel and other resources, and the means for converting evaluation findings into action.

Evaluation necessarily draws attention to our own values and those of others. This is an especially complicated dynamic in interprofessional education, which serves stakeholders who have experienced contrasting forms of professional socialisation. The evaluation of interprofessional education also highlights questions of what is believed to constitute evidence deemed worthy of attention and action (numbers or narrative), and differing conceptions of effectiveness. You may want to refresh your memory of some of these issues with a brief look back at Chapter two.

We have broken down the process of planning a sound evaluation into key areas to be addressed. These should not be seen as sequential stages or even a recipe to be slavishly followed. The usual experience is of addressing many of these aspects in parallel and returning to each in cycles until the full evaluation plan emerges.

Evaluating interprofessional education – why and who for?

Promoting improvement is the ultimate 'why' of any evaluation. This includes specific improvements to the evaluated initiative and, more widely, better informed planning and delivery of interprofessional education at other times and in other places. Thus, providing evidence for action and making suggestions for action is central to the evaluation process. Evaluations are not ends in themselves; they belong to plan-do-study-act cycles of curriculum and evaluation development. Interprofessional education is planned and delivered (Chapters three to eight). Meanwhile, evaluation is planned and conducted (Chapters nine to twelve). Each is subjected to scrutiny with the aim of improvement: the study-act parts of the cycle, applied to the design and implementation of both the interprofessional education and its evaluation. Change is a frequent evaluation-informed action. It is also evaluation-informed action to repeat or continue successful approaches, perhaps evolved from small pilots (as discussed in Chapter five under 'small is beautiful').

The list below provides some indicative examples of why evaluations of interprofessional education may be necessary or advisable. Please take a moment to assess which are applicable in your context and to expand the list in the light of your own concerns, interests and constraints. Evaluations of interprofessional education can, amongst others, do all those things shown in Box 9.1.

Box 9.1   Reasons to evaluate interprofessional education.

- Celebrate and provide evidence of success, perhaps providing exemplars of good practice.
- Measure achievement against specific learning outcomes.
- Identify and contribute to explaining problems that occurred during the development or delivery of an interprofessional learning opportunity; and help find solutions.
- Inform future resource allocation, where resources include direct delivery costs, investment in learning environments and infrastructure, staff development, etc.
- Ensure that the views of those who have little power are heard and considered.
- Formalise and examine intuitive feelings or informal feedback, testing the veracity of these and make more codified knowledge available for rational decision making.

- Inform the integration of interprofessional learning within largely uni-professional curricula.
- Provide clear descriptions of processes and outcomes as a precursor to exploring causal mechanisms and general(isable) principles.
- Compare different approaches to interprofessional education, or compare interprofessional education with uni-professional education.
- Share learning from specific programmes or contexts among the wider communities interested in interprofessional collaboration.
- Satisfy funders that their investment has been used effectively.

The evaluation process involves the collection, sorting and interpretation of a range of information that has a bearing on judgements of effectiveness and other aspects of value. This process is conducted in a manner that is mindful of the needs and interests of (possibly) several different stakeholder groups. The stake-holders for evaluations include all the groups highlighted in Figure 2.2. In fact, many of the questions in that figure are potential evaluation questions.

It is not usually possible for one evaluation to meet the perceived needs of every stakeholder, so evaluations are normally tailored to serve specific groups or specific purposes. The questions listed in Box 9.2 are ones that can help you in this process.

Evaluation scope and boundaries

Sound evaluations are based on the careful delimitation of what is to be evaluated (agreeing the *scope* of the evaluation) and the difficult process of teasing out a

---

Box 9.2   Key questions to tailor your evaluation.

- What do we want to evaluate and why?
- How does this contribute to meeting the needs of various stakeholder groups?
- How will the evaluation findings and interpretations contribute to informed action?
- Who should conduct the evaluation?
- When should the evaluation start and how long should it last?
- What choices and constraints do we have in relation to this evaluation?
- How best can we obtain the data (observations, measurements, narratives, etc.) we require to evaluate the effectiveness of those aspects of the inter-professional education that concern us within this evaluation?
- What resources will be required?
- What will this evaluation *not* attempt to investigate?

manageable list of *relevant and answerable* questions. The evaluator must negotiate the evaluation focus and limits with relevant stakeholders and, particularly for external evaluators, gain an understanding of the context to be evaluated. At this stage the evaluation team may also have an important role in helping several groups of stakeholders to formulate their requirements or aspirations for the evaluation as clearly as possible. This process will probably reveal too many evaluation questions and aims: some of these will conflict. The evaluation team can then assist the stakeholders in prioritising their questions and aims. As part of this process the evaluation team will need to make clear what type of evaluation they can offer; its price and timetable, how this will address the stakeholders' questions and aims, what kind of decisions the evaluation might inform and what limitations the evaluation will have. This careful dialogue will ensure that all parties hold realistic views about what will be evaluated, how this will be done and the anticipated use of the information and insights that are produced. Issues about ownership of information and insights should also be discussed at this stage.

Questions that are specific enough to implicitly suggest how they might be answered are a great advantage in guiding the design and execution of an evaluation. In addition, questions of this type enable readers of your reports to assess very quickly the relevance of your evaluation to their concerns. Suitable questions include:

- What were learners' end-of-course and three-month follow-up reactions to the interprofessional education?
- To what extent did learners' knowledge of the course content improve between time A and time B?
- What auditable changes in practice or service delivery have occurred in the six months following the interprofessional education?
- What forms of interaction and decision making could be observed within interprofessional problem-based learning groups?

Perhaps stop for a moment now, and reflect on the questions you might ask of your interprofessional education: are they specific enough?

Diffuse questions may result in a lack of focus in the evaluation. Breaking them down into two or three focused questions may avert this problem. Examples of diffuse questions include: Did it work? Was it worthwhile?

It is also necessary to be alert to evaluation questions that are focused enough to be answerable only after careful definition of the boundaries to the evaluation, for example: How much did it cost? What have we gained and lost? In each case a range of different conclusions could be reached that is dependent on how widely you 'cast your net' whilst gathering evidence. Thus, it would be necessary to increase the specificity of the evaluation questions by clearly defining boundaries: perhaps a time interval, a particular geographical location, a particular organisational unit, and so on.

The choice of evaluation questions is ultimately a pragmatic one, based on negotiation and the interests of stakeholders in the interprofessional education, the interests and expertise of the evaluators, the resources available and the allocated timeframe. Very few evaluations are comprehensive: a realistic and a worthwhile ambition is a focused study producing credible knowledge and insights that aid improvement in specific ways.

Evaluation types and purpose

Evaluations of educational initiatives are most often categorised as *formative, summative* or *hybrid* (this mirrors categories of assessment, see Chapter six). Formative evaluation is sometimes termed *developmental evaluation* and summative evaluations are sometimes termed *outcomes evaluations*. In essence, formative evaluation examines processes, learning materials and other artefacts (for example, meeting minutes, curriculum documents, feedback forms) and interim outcomes, with a view to providing information and interpretations that can be used to make improvements within the development and delivery phases of an initiative (see Box 9.3). Summative evaluation may examine the same processes, artefacts, and outcomes but with the dual purposes of accounting for the resources used and informing subsequent development and delivery. Summative evaluations should provide evidence and interpretations to help improve the initiative studied, and further, should be presented in ways that allow other initiatives to benefit: thus providing good value for the evaluation resource. As such, formative evaluations usually have a local focus and summative evaluations tend to have local and wider foci.

The distinction between formative and summative evaluation can feel quite blurred in the midst of evaluation activity. The difference between them sometimes amounts only to matters of emphasis and timing. Most evaluations of interprofessional education will be hybrid, containing formative and summative

---

Box 9.3   An example of a formative evaluation.

Cornish *et al.* (2003) described a formative evaluation of an innovative inter-professional course that employed video-conferencing technology for mental health practitioners working in remote rural locations in Canada. The course allowed 34 practitioners from a range of professions including medicine, nursing and social work to participate in presentations and discussions on issues linked to the care of patients with mental health problems.

To help understand the impact of the course, questionnaires and interviews were collected from all participants. In addition, field notes were gathered that tracked participants' responses and interactions as well as the technical performance of the video-conferencing equipment.

(Continues)

Findings from the evaluation revealed that participants enjoyed their inter-professional learning experience. They also reported that their understanding of each other's professional roles had been enhanced, and that there was increased interprofessional cohesion and support between members of this group. Despite generally high levels of satisfaction with the use of video-conferencing technology for the course, participants found the reliability of the equipment was, on occasions, poor.

Based on the findings from this formative evaluation, the authors stated that following a number of refinements to the technology, they aimed to expand this interprofessional programme to other health and social care practitioners located in rural settings.

elements. The balance between formative and summative evaluation may shift as the interprofessional initiative matures, or it may be more cyclical in nature.

There are many approaches to evaluation reflecting different cultures and preferences (for example, disciplinary culture, professional culture, organisa-tional culture, national culture). Therefore, evaluations of interprofessional edu-cation adopt many different approaches, as the boxed examples within this book show. Descriptive or interpretive qualitative and mixed methods evaluations predominate, most often presented as case studies. Boxes 9.4 and 9.5 demonstrate this. Experimental approaches focusing on largely quantifiable outcomes of inter-professional education are relatively rare but Box 9.6 provides an example.

Box 9.4   An interpretative evaluation.

Alderson *et al.* (2002) describe the qualitative evaluation of the impact of 11 interprofessional ethics seminars for hospital-based staff in the UK. Fifty-six staff from a range of clinical specialities (including obstetrics, neonatal and haematological care) and a variety of professional groups (including medi-cine, nursing, midwifery and psychology) participated in one or more of these sessions.

The seminars aimed to improve participants' interprofessional understand-ing of ethical dilemmas related to the social and ethical consequences of advances in genetics and their impact on policy and health care practice.

Qualitative data were collected in two phases. Initially, to ensure that each of the seminars was well targeted to meet the needs of staff, in-depth face-to-face and telephone interviews were conducted with 70 members of staff. To evaluate the impact of the sessions on the participants, follow-up interviews were also undertaken.

It was found that participants enjoyed the sessions. In addition, they felt that they improved their understanding of ethical dilemmas and their know-ledge of the roles of colleagues from other professions.

Box 9.5   A mixed-method evaluation.

Barnes *et al.* (2000) report a mixed-method evaluation of a part-time interprofessional programme for community mental health practitioners in England. The course led to a postgraduate certificate, diploma or Master's degree in community mental health (depending on the length of study) and was open to nurses, occupational therapists, social workers, psychologists and psychiatrists. Service users contributed to the management of the course and the evaluation.

Quantitative data (questionnaires) and qualitative data (interviews, observations) were gathered to comprehensively identify the impact of the course on participants' understanding of their professional roles and their attitudes towards one another. While questionnaire and interview data assessed course outcomes, the observational data focused on exploring the processes of interaction between learners during the course.

Questionnaire data collected at the end of the first and second year of study on the programme revealed that although participants' understanding of roles had improved, the course did not alter their professional allegiances or stereotypes. Small group interviews revealed that participants valued the mix of different professional groups on the course, but felt that there was insufficient time to get to know each other. Observations of the interprofessional sessions revealed that tutors spent little time focused on helping participants understand issues connected to interprofessional collaboration.

Box 9.6   An experimental evaluation, UK.

Thompson *et al.* (2000) undertook a randomised-controlled trial to evaluate the impact on patient care of implementing a clinical practice guideline for the treatment of depression within general practice. Fifty-nine general practices were recruited into the trial. Practices were computer randomised to the initiative group (made up from 29 teams of general practitioners and practice nurses) who received interprofessional sessions on the guideline, or to a control group (made up from 30 teams) who did not receive these sessions until completion of the trial.

To assess the impact of the new guideline, questionnaires were distributed to the initiative and control group participants before and after the delivery of the interprofessional sessions. In addition, depression scale scores of patients treated by the practitioners in both groups were collected, as well as data on practitioners' ability to recognise depression. To examine the longer-term impact of the guideline, follow-up data were collected after six months.

(Continues)

It was found that the new guideline was well received by participants. In addition, 80% of participants felt their management of depression had improved as a result of introducing the guideline. However, depression scale scores and depression detection rates did not alter significantly between the initiative and control groups following the interprofessional education, or at the six-month follow-up stage of the trial.

Some evaluations provide an external perspective; others are collaboratively constructed, as evaluators and participants build a mutual understanding of what is occurring (e.g. action research projects); yet others comprise reflective insider accounts. We will say more about insider and outsider evaluation in Chapter ten.

Evaluation paradigms, methodologies and methods

All evaluations are shaped and influenced by the values, theories and concepts of the disciplines and/or professions of those involved in the work. Another way of saying this is that evaluations are set within a particular *paradigm* or way of thinking about the world. The ways in which evidence is created and acknowledged as valid in a particular paradigm (worldview) is often very different to that in other paradigms. The nature of the relationship between evaluators and the evaluated context also differs between paradigms. These differences in turn influence how enquiries to establish evidence (methodologies) should proceed.

A methodology, or theory of how an inquiry proceeds, analyses assumptions, principles and procedures. For example, it defines what forms a researchable problem, what constitutes legitimate evidence-based explanation and how generalisability should be viewed. To do this the evaluator needs methods, which can also be thought of as procedures, techniques or strategies. So, for example, experimental and quasi-experimental inquiry, ethnography and phenomenology are all theoretical ways of enquiring into the impact, effectiveness or role of something in the world: they are methodologies. In contrast, controlled trials, participant observation and interviewing are methods: processes undertaken to collect data for interpretation.

Particular clusters of methods tend to be associated with each methodological approach, but the same method, particularly observation and interviewing, can be used very differently, depending on the evaluator's methodological stance. This, in turn, is influenced by the underlying evaluation paradigm. The most usual paradigm classification for evaluation work is to view the fundamental influences on methodology and method as either positivist, interpretive or change-orientated.

Sound, fit-for-purpose evaluations can be very conservative or highly innovative in terms of their methodology and methods of data collection and analysis. It is the quality of thinking and planning that determines the soundness of the evaluation design. The conduct of the evaluation process then determines the quality of the evaluation findings. Naturally, the evaluation design should be matched to the expertise of the evaluator(s) and the available resources.

When you plan an evaluation of interprofessional education remember to examine your emergent evaluation design for congruence between methodology and methods:

- Ask yourself whether these plans contain implicit methodological assumptions, associated with a particular paradigm.
- Take time to bring to the surface any buried assumptions. This allows scrutiny of their necessity and sufficiency, and helps identify any contradictions.
- Look carefully at your evaluation questions and ask whether your chosen methodology is appropriate to address these questions.
- Then examine your chosen methods of data collection and data analysis to check their fit with the evaluation questions and methodology.

The following sections briefly consider some methodological approaches within each paradigm that could be useful for the evaluation of your interprofessional education initiative. Additional descriptions of these and other evaluation approaches can be found within the books listed in the further reading section at the end of this chapter.

Change orientated evaluation: action research

The action-research approach involves a spiral of interlocking cycles of planning, acting, observing and reflecting. Action researchers work collaboratively with participants to clarify development needs, design and implement initiatives, and evaluate processes and outcomes. There is a commitment to careful documenting of the process. This permits analysis and the formation of new insights that will be shared with the wider community through a programme of dissemination to audiences beyond the immediate action research site(s). Terms you may have heard that relate to the action research approach include plan-do-study-act (PDSA) cycles of quality improvement and 'double loop learning' (Argyris, 1990). Box 9.7 describes an action-research study of interprofessional practice development with interprofessional education, where the planned practice development had a disappointing outcome but may have stimulated very important interprofessional learning.

The strengths of action research lie in advancing theoretical knowledge and adding to the relevant evidence base *simultaneously with* solving practical problems in real settings. Participating practitioners gain a deeper understanding of practice and are empowered to improve it. There are many approaches to action research, for example Hart & Bond (1995, pp. 38–48) proposed a typology comprising experimental, organisational, professionalising and empowering forms, and discussed classifications proposed by others. Certain approaches to action research have been criticised for privileging groups over individuals and it has been suggested that, through overemphasising rational consensus, action research

---

Box 9.7   An action-research study, UK.

Atwal (2002) described an action-research study undertaken on an orthopaedic ward in an inner-city teaching hospital. The study focused on the development, implementation and evaluation of a new interprofessional discharge guideline designed to enhance the efficiency of discharge and the quality of patient care.

An interprofessional action-research group, led by the author and consisting of doctors, nurses, occupational therapists and social workers, was formed to begin designing the discharge guideline. An important part of the planning stage of the group's work was a Delphi survey carried out with staff to obtain a consensus opinion for the design of the guideline.

The action research group implemented the guideline by producing discharge documentation that outlined the new discharge procedure. They also offered a series of interprofessional training sessions to ward staff to help them understand how the guideline should operate.

Questionnaire, interview and observational data were gathered to evaluate the impact of the new discharge guideline. Results were disappointing. It was found that the new guideline was largely unused by staff as most found it too time consuming to employ. Indeed, it was found that the guideline actually worsened interprofessional relations because differences of opinion around its use resulted in friction between staff. Despite these disappointments, the author noted that the staff involved in the study began to think more critically about how they collaborate in practice.

---

can encourage conservative solutions. For an extended discussion on the spectrum of action-research approaches and strengths and weaknesses, we recommend Hart & Bond (1995, Part I) and Cohen *et al.* (2000, Chapter thirteen).

The evaluator undertaking an action research approach acts as facilitator, guide, summariser, formulator (of ideas, questions and interpretations for discussion) and also has a role in raising issues that might be otherwise overlooked. This demands a very high level of interpersonal skill and diligence in the time consuming tasks of record keeping and background research.

Other methodologies suitable for initiating and supporting change include appreciative enquiry (Hammond, 1998), change laboratory (Engeström, 1999), organisational learning[1] (Argyris, 1990) and solutions focus (Jackson & McKergow, 2002).

Interpretive evaluation: illuminative and responsive methodologies

Illuminative evaluation (Parlett, 1981) is an approach that aims to describe and interpret practices, influential factors, outcomes and problems *that are meaningful*

---

[1] Continuous quality improvement (CQI) and total quality management (TQM) are processes that use organisational learning theory.

and important to the stakeholders of interprofessional education in a specific context. It allows unexpected issues or outcomes to be identified. It usually requires the presentation of multiple perspectives.

Stake (1975) coined the term 'responsive evaluation'; in many respects this is similar to illuminative evaluation. Stake encouraged us to think of three types of stakeholder: agents, beneficiaries and victims (an example of a victim might be a person whose workload increases dramatically as a result of a newly introduced interprofessional education initiative, who does not receive adequate recognition or assistance). This reminds us of the criteria for effectiveness that we set out at the beginning of Chapter two: that (on balance) outcomes should be positive, at acceptable cost and without unacceptable side effects. The inadvertent creation of a group of victims might be viewed as an unacceptable side effect.

Illuminative evaluation takes the form of case study research, sharing the strengths and weaknesses of that approach. Case studies present an accessible authentic description that can accommodate complexity, nuance and the unanticipated. Case study is a manageable evaluation design for a single evaluator, although case study data can quickly reach unmanageable proportions, then proving difficult to organise for presentation and interpretation. The degree to which case study findings and interpretations are generalisable is debatable. There may be concerns about the influence of the evaluator on the evaluation outcomes, despite attention to reflexivity. For a useful guide to case study approaches we recommend Gomm *et al.* (2000).

Other forms of evaluation that normally belong to the interpretive paradigm include those that draw from methodologies such as ethnography, grounded theory, interpretive interactionism and phenomenology. These and other qualitative methodologies are presented at varying levels of detail and rigour in a large number of specialised and more general research or evaluation texts. For a concise but rigorous series of overviews we recommend dipping into Denzin & Lincoln (2000), or volumes one and two of the same work in paperback form (Denzin & Lincoln 1998; Denzin & Lincoln 2003).

Positivist approach: quasi-experimental outcome evaluation

Full experimental evaluation designs involve the random allocation of participants to control and intervention groups to permit comparison of outcomes (in this case interprofessional education would be the intervention). Two common experimental designs are randomised controlled trial (RCT, Box 9.6 above) and controlled before and after (CBA) study. Experimental studies are rarely undertaken to evaluate interprofessional education, often because there is no suitable control group, or because randomisation cannot be agreed with stakeholders. Some would also argue that experimental designs are rarely appropriate given the type of questions we have about the effectiveness of interprofessional education. However, a quasi-experimental approach is a little more common. Comparison groups are constructed that as closely as possible match the experimental group (interprofessional education participants) in terms of characteristics that may be associated with outcomes. Rossi *et al.* (2004) provided a good description of this approach.

When it is not possible to construct a separate control group 'reflexive controls' may be used: these are observations made before the interprofessional education commenced. Such before-and-after designs are relatively common in the evaluation of interprofessional education and Box 9.8 provides an example.

Experimental and quasi-experimental approaches are robust means of detecting the net effects of initiatives, in our case interprofessional education, but they have little to say about the mechanisms that mediate the net effects. This highlights the need to match carefully the evaluation methodology and evaluation questions. We will look more closely at evaluation questions in the next section.

The potency of experimental and quasi-experimental designs depends on the strength of the control element and the strength of the sampling that is achieved. This may mean that an initiative is not studied in its natural state and that results from evaluations of this type may be difficult to replicate in other real world settings.

Box 9.8   A before-and-after study.

Schreiber *et al.* (2002) reported a before-and-after study in the USA that evaluated a one-month interprofessional course for army teams of surgeons, nurses, emergency medical technicians and operating room technicians. The course was based in a non-army setting (a large general hospital) and aimed to enhance the practitioners' approach to the treatment and care of trauma patients.

The course was offered in three stages. Initially, in profession-specific groups, practitioners were introduced to the roles, duties, procedures and protocols of their civilian counterparts. Second, practitioners were offered interprofessional sessions in which they undertook general surgical procedures and emergency resuscitations. Finally, each of the army teams worked together in the emergency centre of the hospital covering night shifts for the civilian practitioners.

To assess the effect of this course on each of the teams, questionnaire data were collected before and after the course. A comparison of pre-course and post-course questionnaires revealed that participants' experience of working together in the hospital resulted in the teams obtaining greater exposure to trauma cases than they had received at their army base. Consequently, it was found that all participants reported a significant increase in their confidence of collaborating together as an interprofessional trauma team.

Given the lack of peacetime trauma experience for military teams, the authors concluded that interprofessional trauma training in civilian settings can assist these practitioners in their clinical practice.

Positivist evaluation: cost-benefit analysis

An economic evaluation of interprofessional education would try to enumerate the resources that it had consumed and would probably compare these with related cost savings, income generation or other benefits. This is quite a complex task. Some costs and benefits are straightforward to identify, for example staff time, rooms used, advertising, administrative service time, provision of learning materials, IT support, learner fees, travel and subsistence costs and so on. But interprofessional education, just like other forms of education, is a complex activity. It is a long-term investment that spans a number of organisations. There are many possible costs and benefits that are much harder to identify.

Since interprofessional education is about improving collaboration, the quality of care and working lives, benefits might conceivably include: minimising duplication of effort and hence costs; more effective and hence shorter episodes of care; improved recruitment and lower attrition of staff and students; and fewer mistakes with their associated costs. Costs might include: increased administrative overheads because inter-organisational working involves coping with systems that are not fully aligned; higher consumption of services as referral or involvement becomes better established, easier and largely expected.

The number of elements to be weighed within an economic evaluation increases rapidly as one moves out in time and space from the actual delivery of the interprofessional education. Boundaries must be drawn sufficiently wide to form a coherent picture without forgetting that this picture will be partial, for example costs and benefits within one organisation, for one service, for a particular client group, or within a particular time interval. It should, nevertheless, be remembered that economic evaluations that employ cost-effectiveness or cost-benefit analyses tend to overlook features of an initiative or context that are difficult to express in monetary terms.

Formal cost–benefit analysis of interprofessional education initiatives is very rare. When authors examine the economic impact of an interprofessional initiative, they tend to do so by focusing on fiscal outcomes. For example, in their evaluation of the introduction of an interprofessional clinical guideline for the care of pneumonia, Gottlieb *et al.* (1996) found that the new guideline contributed to a reduction of the average cost of care per patient episode. Pryce and Reeves (1997) compared the costs of profession-specific provision of a community-based module for first-year undergraduate dental, medical and nursing students with the costs of interprofessional provision, and found that marginal cost savings were achieved by the interprofessional provision.

On rare occasions, authors will collect both fiscal and clinical outcome data. While these evaluations do not employ a formal cost–benefit or cost-effectiveness analysis, they help provide a more comprehensive insight into the possible costs and benefits to patient care of interprofessional education. For example, Price *et al.* (1999) found that following the implementation of an interprofessional guideline for infection control within a surgical setting, patient care costs were reduced without a reduction in the quality of patient outcomes.

Returning to presage, process and product

In Chapter three we spent some time considering aspects of presage, process and product in relation to interprofessional education. The concepts *presage*, *process* and *product* form a useful checklist to test your contextual understanding of the interprofessional education you will evaluate. They may also provide a convenient structure within your evaluation design. Perhaps take a moment to look back at Figure 3.1.

Presage factors are influences and constraints on the design and delivery of interprofessional education. Presage alone is rarely the subject of evaluation, but key presage factors may need to be mapped to enable appreciation of realised delivery and outcomes. Thus, even when their main focus is elsewhere, evaluators should be alert to the influences of presage factors.

Process, within the 3P model, is concerned with the delivery of the interprofessional education. A process evaluation would focus on interaction, decision making, approaches to learning and teaching, levels of engagement, and so on. These are important because effective processes aid the achievement of effective outcomes. Evaluating processes within interprofessional education will strengthen the pedagogy (underpinning conception of teaching and learning) in interprofessional education. At the time of writing, no pure process evaluations of interprofessional education could be located in the literature. Where authors do report the processes that occur within an interprofessional education initiative, outcome data are always reported in far more detail. For example, while evaluations by both Roberts *et al.* (2000) and Fallsberg & Hammar (2000) provided insights into the interprofessional interactions that occur between pre-qualification students, both papers were more heavily weighted in favour of reporting the outcomes produced by their respective initiatives. Such a bias may be inevitable: in health and social care effectiveness is usually couched in terms of outcomes and processes can sometimes be overlooked until they begin to produce unwelcome outcomes.

Product, within the 3P model, is concerned with the outcomes of the interprofessional education. An outcomes evaluation would focus on one or more of the categories in Table 2.1. which we will discuss further in Chapter eleven. Most published evaluations of interprofessional education focus on outcomes: Box 9.9 provides an example.

Usually evaluations of interprofessional education emphasise short-term outcomes because longer-term outcomes are somewhat complicated to capture and increasing the duration of an evaluation usually increases costs. Longitudinal evaluation designs allow repeated observation of the phenomena or variables that may be influenced by interprofessional education. This is helpful, but inevitably limited because professional practice is highly complex and influenced by many factors besides interprofessional education.

An exclusive focus on outcomes evaluation would not explore the mechanisms linking interprofessional education to its outcomes (positive or negative) and would overlook the supportive or inhibitory nature of a host of presage and

---

Box 9.9   An outcomes-based evaluation.

Bluespruce *et al.* (2001) report an outcomes evaluation of an interprofessional course that aimed to improve health and social care practitioners' attitudes towards an understanding of human immunodeficiency virus (HIV). Forty-nine health and social care staff from two primary care clinics based in a large managed care organisation in the USA took part in the programme. Participants included doctors, nurses and social workers.

Participants were initially offered four interprofessional sessions in which they undertook team discussions, role-plays and patient case stories. To help reinforce the learning from the sessions, participants were offered written materials (e.g. HIV risk management protocols), 'on-the-job' team support, and two further interactive sessions.

The authors measured the following outcomes: changes in participants' attitudes towards HIV, and knowledge and skills of the management of the virus. Questionnaires were distributed to participants both before and after the delivery of the programme. Findings revealed that participants' attitudes towards HIV had significantly improved following their involvement in this interprofessional programme. In addition, participants reported significant improvements in terms of their knowledge, confidence and skills of working with HIV-positive patients.

---

process influences. This would make it difficult to decide on the actions that should follow from the evaluation findings. Evaluation-informed action is stronger if there is a balance between process and outcome evaluation.

Conclusion

Evaluations of interprofessional education systematically record processes and outcomes, providing thoughtful interpretations of these to increase stakeholders' understanding and to enable judgements of value. Evaluations help people make more informed decisions and promote improvement.

Evaluators should try to work in partnership with representatives of each stakeholder group during the planning of the evaluation. Answerable and useful evaluation questions need to be negotiated with stakeholders and, in addition, all parties should be clear about things that the evaluation will not address.

There are many different types of evaluation, each having strengths and weaknesses in relation to particular questions and particular contexts. Sound, fit-for-purpose evaluations can be very conservative or highly innovative. The complexity of the evaluation process needs to be tailored to the expertise and resources available. It is the quality of thinking and planning that determines the soundness of the evaluation design, so time invested at this stage pays dividends.

Fundamental decisions include: the purpose and audience(s) for an evaluation; the evaluation questions; selecting an appropriate methodological perspective and, following this, an appropriate design with appropriate methods; the balance between formative and summative evaluation; and the balance between process and outcome evaluation.

Key points

- Informed actions (including informed no change) are the important outcomes of evaluation.
- Evaluation-informed action is stronger if there is a balance between process and outcome evaluation.
- Evaluation questions should reflect the concerns of stakeholders and need to be refined until they are answerable.
- Evaluation questions can be addressed through a variety of methodological approaches, suggesting a variety of evaluation designs and the use of a wide range of methods, all needing to be matched to available expertise and resources.

Further reading

Blaikie, N. (2000) *Designing Social Research: the Logic of Anticipation*. Polity Press, Cambridge.

Clarke, A. & Dawson, R. (1999) *Evaluation Research: an Introduction to Principles, Methods and Practice*. Sage, London.

Cohen, L., Manion, L. & Morrison, K. (2000) *Research Methods in Education*. 5th edn. Routledge Falmer, London.

Pope, C. & Mays, N. (1999) *Qualitative Research in Health Care*, (revised edition). BMJ Books, London.

Reason, P. & Bradbury, H. (2000) *The Handbook of Action Research: Participative Inquiry and Practice*. Sage, London.

Rossi, P., Lipsey, M. & Freeman, H. (2004) *Evaluation: a Systematic Approach*. 7th edn. Sage, Newbury Park, California.

Tashakkori, A. & Teddlie, C. (2002) *Handbook of Mixed Methods in Social and Behavioural Research*. Sage, London.

Yin, R. (2003) *Case Study Research: Design and Methods*. 3rd edn. Sage, London.

10 Developing Sound Evaluations

Introduction

Having considered the fundamental decisions that begin the process of planning and conducting a sound evaluation of interprofessional education, we now turn our attention to a second layer of concepts and issues. These influence actions, choices and, ultimately, the effectiveness of evaluations of interprofessional education.

Evaluation as exchange

The evaluation of interprofessional education can be viewed as an exchange between partners. This is both an ethical and a practical stance that enhances the commitment of all stakeholders to the successful completion of the evaluation. Evaluators bring a range of technical expertise and knowledge of other contexts to the evaluation endeavour: outsider evaluators also bring fresh eyes, ears and ideas. We will say more about insider and outsider evaluation a little later in this chapter. The evaluators' expertise and perspectives are exchanged with participants' insider knowledge and interpretations of the interprofessional education. Through this process new understanding can be generated that can be applied to the development of the interprofessional education. These new understandings may also contribute more widely to perspectives on the processes and outcomes of developing, delivering and evaluating interprofessional education.

Organisations and managers commission and facilitate evaluations because in exchange they gain recognition from their involvement, and new knowledge or perspectives to inform strategic and operational planning. Patients, clients, learners, tutors, curriculum developers and other participants contribute to evaluations because in exchange they gain a platform for their views and hope for improvements affecting themselves or those that follow. If the evaluation is appropriately designed participants may also gain professional or personal development from their involvement, and intrinsic satisfaction. In exchange for their professional expertise evaluators gain recognition for their work, personal and professional development, and intrinsic satisfaction from contributing to a well-executed evaluation that promotes positive developments. All parties give important resources and perspectives to evaluations and all parties should be able to take away developmental outcomes.

Governance and ethics

Evaluations of interprofessional education must be conducted ethically and with due regard for the governance procedures operating in different contexts. People are the focus of education, so virtually all educational evaluation and research is human-subjects research. Unless you confine yourself to a formative evaluation for the course team only, you are highly likely to need to seek approval for your evaluation from a research ethics committee, and also to register the evaluation with the research and development offices of participating organisations. This may need to be repeated if unforeseen circumstances or unexpected initial findings necessitate changes to your evaluation plan or timetable.

When formulating your evaluation plan it is helpful to pause intermittently and review it for ethical concerns by asking questions such as:

- What does informed consent mean in this context?
- How are participants going to be kept informed of the ongoing evaluation processes and emergent findings?
- How will initial consent to participate in the evaluation be recorded and how will ongoing consent be checked?
- Might any aspects of the evaluation plan feel coercive?
- What level of confidentiality and anonymity can be assured and how will this be achieved?
- Does the evaluation team have sufficient expertise to conduct this evaluation competently and sensitively?
- Is this evaluation designed to reveal new things that have practical significance?

Perhaps take a few moments to add additional questions that are pertinent to your own contexts.

Insider and outsider evaluation

An insider evaluator may be regarded as a person who is immersed in the development and delivery of interprofessional education and also undertakes an evaluation of one or more facets of that interprofessional education. An outside evaluator is, at least to some degree, external to the context to be evaluated. A fully independent external evaluator has no allegiance to any of the participating organisations, but it is fairly uncommon for this to happen. More often an evaluator or small evaluation team is employed by one of the participating organisations. Their role is to conduct evaluation to support the development and delivery of the interprofessional education without, themselves, bearing primary responsibility for the development and delivery activities. Just as we noted in respect of the boundaries between formative and summative evaluation, the boundary between insider and outsider evaluation can sometimes feel quite blurred in practice, depending on the stage of the evaluation and on its methodological approach. Participatory approaches, such as action research, specifically seek to minimise the separation of insider and outsider evaluation.

Insider evaluators gain from an established preliminary understanding of the evaluation context, although they need strong reflexive skills to guard against inadequate separation between their preconceived ideas and the emerging evaluation findings. Insider evaluators may find negotiating access to people, places and documents is eased by their known insider status. On the other hand, outsider evaluators may obtain more candid feedback from participants since there would be less concern about internal politics or hurting the evaluator's feelings. Insider evaluators may be able to feed their emergent evaluation understandings into the development cycle more quickly and effectively than outsider evaluators. However, outsider evaluators are necessarily allocated time and other resources with which to conduct their evaluation. Insider evaluators may be expected to incorporate this work within already pressed schedules and stretched resources. There is a greater risk that insider evaluation will be curtailed or delayed, as urgent and equally important issues relating to development and delivery crowd in.

A useful option is to seek a balance between insider and outsider evaluation, perhaps employing a part-time outsider who combines the role of evaluator and adviser. This has resource implications and we will elaborate on resources a little later.

Securing sufficient preliminary understanding

Sufficient familiarisation with the context to be evaluated and the work of others is essential at the planning stage if oversights are to be avoided. Try to see this as the beginning of an ongoing process. Your work will be of a higher quality if you continue to listen, read and think throughout the evaluation process, allowing your evolving knowledge to influence the fine tuning of your evaluation and to inform your interpretations of the findings.

The local context

Evaluators continually develop their understanding of the context to be evaluated, but essential groundwork for preparing an appropriate and viable evaluation plan includes a substantial investment in listening, observing and reading. This is most obviously true for outsider evaluators but remains true for insiders.

Even insider evaluators, immersed in the development and delivery of the inter-professional education, will hold a partial view of presage and process factors as they affect people from the different participating professions and other stake-holder groups.

Information-gathering conversations with people closely involved with the interprofessional education from different perspectives are very important. Out-sider evaluators may be permitted to observe meetings or even groups engaged in interprofessional learning. Insider evaluators may find themselves more con-sciously adopting the role of participant observer. In these situations it is import-ant to announce your presence and its purpose, checking for unease or objections. For example, you might state that you are a potential evaluator of this interpro-fessional education programme, trying to increase your understanding of the programme and making notes to inform the design of any evaluation. It is too soon to apply for ethical committee approval for your evaluation so you need to remember that you will not be collecting data or piloting instruments at this stage.

Reading is another important aspect of understanding the context. The documents generated by the interprofessional education initiative and its partici-pant organisations will greatly increase your understanding of the context to be evaluated.

Whilst developing your preliminary understanding of the local context you may be lucky enough to discover that earlier work has resulted in the creation of important baseline data. For example, routine record keeping might include a database of demographic and other characteristics for interprofessional education participants (for example age, ethnicity, prior educational experience and qualifica-tions, subsequent educational and career trajectories). Although access to existing data sets is not always straightforward because of the need to safeguard personal and sensitive information, there may be ways to negotiate the release of anonymous or summary data for use in your evaluation. In contexts where an adequate baseline data set exists, against which subsequent change related to interprofessional education can be evaluated, evaluation can be quicker and less costly.

The wider context

Continuing with the processes of reading, listening and discussing, it is also important to familiarise yourself with the wider context of relevant policy initia-tives and examples of other evaluations of interprofessional education. The com-munity of interprofessional education evaluators is continually drawing from knowledge developed in other fields, and innovating, developing and testing improved evaluation designs and means of gathering evidence. Methodically searching the available literature, including reviews such as that reported in our companion volume (Barr *et al.*, 2005), allows you to benefit from the insights and developments of those that precede you and prevents unnecessary replication of basic work. The publishing process means that there can be a delay of many months before key work is easily accessible in journals and books. To be familiar with the most current developments in the evaluation of interprofessional education it may be necessary to attend professional meetings, to join networks that host meetings or electronic discussions, and to search websites.

Throughout the information gathering process, aimed at securing a sufficient preliminary understanding to yield a sound evaluation plan, you will be judging the relevance and quality of what you read and hear. This is a matter of professional judgement, but checking whether material has been peer reviewed can be helpful.

Finally, studying evaluation methodology and methods is a further aspect of securing sufficient preliminary understanding to inform the development of a sound evaluation plan for your interprofessional education.

Negotiating access

Assessing and negotiating access are a central part of evaluation planning. If you wish to collect data from students, patients or clients, or to collect data in educational or clinical settings, there will be several gate-keepers who will have to agree to allow you access to 'their' students, clients or practice settings. Normally, such negotiation has to precede gaining ethical approval for your evaluation, since evidence of support from key gate-keepers will be required for such approval.

We mentioned naturally occurring data archives in the previous section. Negotiating access to fairly public records, such as committee minutes, or access to anonymised records, may be relatively straightforward. Access to key strategic documents and individual records that were compiled for other reasons will be rather more complicated, often requiring the design of mechanisms for obtaining informed consent from those to whom the records refer.

Negotiation of access to places, people and records does not end when the study begins. Maintaining ongoing access is a continuing process requiring evaluators to draw on their professional judgement and interpersonal skills. Job changes are frequent in health and social care. This may mean the departure of well-briefed and supportive gate-keepers and the arrival of gate-keepers in need of briefing. New gate-keepers may bring different perspectives, priorities and concerns; and continued access cannot be assumed. Your evaluation plan may need to be reviewed and revised.

The evaluation plan

The multiple streams of planning that we are discussing in Section III will converge in a plan for your evaluation. The plan should be recorded in a document so that the intended form and progress of the evaluation is available for scrutiny, to consult as a guide to action, and as a historical artefact. The evaluation plan is likely to form a contract between the evaluation team and any funding body, also between the evaluators and participating organisations. The evaluation plan, together with relevant codes of professional conduct, guides the individual contracts that are made between each evaluator and each participating individual. The content of an evaluation plan reflects its multiple purposes.

An evaluation plan will address: the agreed purposes and scope of the evaluation (including anticipated limitations); the evaluation question(s); justification of the methodological approach; details of data collection methods; a data analysis plan; a dissemination plan; resources required; roles and responsibilities of each member of the evaluation team and other key individuals; the evaluation timetable; ethical considerations; quality mechanisms; and perhaps a risk assessment for the study.

Plan carefully and still expect change

Careful and rigorous planning is a very important underpinning for a successful evaluation. Unfortunately, pre-planning is not sufficient to ensure success. Evaluation contexts are complex and a certain degree of unpredictability is inevitable. Regular reviews of the context and the evaluation's progress, combined with a willingness to replan, are necessary survival skills. Common changes that buffet evaluations include: policy changes, departure of key gate-keepers or champions, loss of resources, changes to the interprofessional education during the period of evaluation, and the appearance of new or previously hidden agendas. These changes tend to be more of a problem in long-term studies, experimental or quasi-experimental studies, and outcome evaluations that lack any process or developmental strand; and for inexperienced evaluators. More experienced evaluators become more adept (although it never feels sufficiently adept) at predicting trouble ahead and formulating 'Plan B'. One means of feeling less alone when grappling with changes influencing your evaluation is to read the 'changes' or 'limitations' sections of other evaluation reports. Here, authors will often describe the circumstances and rationale for plans and revised plans. Not only can this provide some comfort as you change your plans, but, read in advance, can prepare you for changes you might need to make to your enquiry.

Policy

Policy at all levels, from national government to local management, can influence the form and provision of interprofessional education. Policy makers depart and arrive; even those that remain in post unpredictably begin to pursue new ideas or priorities. Your perfectly planned evaluation may need revision in the light of one large or several small policy changes. The nature of interprofessional education is that it spans organisations, increasing the likelihood of being affected by policy change. In addition, interprofessional education is a long-term investment and your evaluation may be planned to follow-up participating individuals and organisations over many months or even years, thus increasing exposure to policy and organisational changes.

Gate-keepers and champions

Passage of time increases the likelihood of changes among the evaluation's gate-keepers and champions. We discussed champions in the context of planning and developing interprofessional education in Chapter four. These are the people with whom you will have negotiated access to various members of staff, places and artefacts; and have agreed the terms and conditions for that access. They are also the people who are likely to support your evaluation within the review and decision-making structures of their organisations. Gate-keepers and champions will help you to secure evaluation resources, perhaps funds, but more likely and equally useful, the loan of certain equipment, places for evaluators to work while data collecting, access to staff canteens, cloakrooms and libraries, assistance with security procedures, and so on. The departure of a gate-keeper may stall your evaluation. The arrival of a new gate-keeper may mean changes to negotiated arrangements, ranging from minor adjustments, through requests for new evaluation priorities, up to complete loss of access.

Loss of resources

Once secured, resources associated with an evaluation contract (for example funds and equipment) are unlikely to be lost, although sometimes the release of funds for later stages of an evaluation is made subject to successful completion and reporting of earlier stages. But informally negotiated resources, for example the use of desk space or photocopying facilities in fieldwork settings, are more vulnerable to loss. This makes it especially important that the evaluation contract should secure all the resources that are essential for conducting the evaluation.

Informally negotiated resources can make a huge difference to the smooth running and efficiency of the evaluation, and to the quality of life of evaluators. This makes it important to remain alert to the impact of the evaluation in the interprofessional education settings and to be alert to changes that may impact on the evaluation. A proactive offer to modify your use of informally negotiated resources may avert their loss if it transpires that the evaluation and the core business of the fieldwork site begin to conflict.

People are by far the most important evaluation resources. Short-term evaluation contracts and the portfolio nature of evaluation careers, in addition to the initiative of other major life events, means that evaluations of interprofessional education sometimes lose key staff at critical moments. This will necessitate urgent review of achievements to date against the evaluation plan, to formulate an honest appraisal of what might now be possible. Early communication with key representatives of the range of evaluation stakeholders is very important. It maintains goodwill and confidence in the evaluation team, and may generate surprising new ideas and offers of assistance.

The criminal (theft, vandalism) or natural disaster (fire, flood) varieties of loss of resources are always possible, although thankfully rare. The best safeguard is diligent back-up record keeping, ideally every day, combined with secure storage away from the main evaluation site.

Changes to the interprofessional education

Evaluation plans are made in relation to the anticipated delivery of interprofessional education during the agreed evaluation period. Then many things may change, including:

- The timing, frequency and capacity of the interprofessional education programme
- The means of selecting or allocating learners or staff
- Approaches to teaching or providing learning resources
- Policy imperatives or the actions of key stakeholders may modify the aims and objectives of the interprofessional education
- Different professions, organisations and care contexts may join or leave the initiative

Any of these changes could render certain aspects of the evaluation plan obsolete or leave it with inadequate coverage. Replanning will become inevitable and may necessitate a return to the committees that granted approval for the evaluation in order that they can scrutinise the changed plans.

Insider evaluators will probably have naturally occurring knowledge of organisational and curriculum changes. Outsider evaluators need to establish mechanisms for keeping up with changes of this type. This might be achieved by, for example, gaining observer status on the interprofessional education steering group, or through a schedule of regular meetings with a key contact(s). You may like to take a few moments to consider the possibilities for keeping abreast of influential changes in your own context.

We should remember that changes to the interprofessional education do not always represent an inconvenience to the evaluation plan. Developmental evaluations and, in particular, action-research studies, seek to support informed change. The design of these evaluations includes flexibility to respond to emergent areas of activity. Changes to the interprofessional education are often included among the evaluation's successes.

New or previously hidden agendas

Education and evaluation are both politically charged processes, capable of precipitating change and evoking emotion, susceptible to misuse and subversion. Commissioning or accepting an evaluation can be:

- An act driven by a desire for greater understanding or conversely, as a mechanism for confirming existing views
- A means to promote change or to stave off change for a while

- A means to reward or punish people's efforts
- A way to promote evidence-based practice or to pay lip service to this agenda
- Aimed at promoting or undermining interprofessional education

Some pre-existing agendas may be kept hidden from the evaluation team, emerging later and hampering the progress of the evaluation. It is not uncommon for various stakeholders to have different (and probably conflicting) agendas for the implementation of the evaluation. Although, as we discussed earlier, evaluators will seek sufficient preliminary understanding of the local context to permit the emergence of a sound evaluation plan, the amount of preliminary work that can be undertaken is necessarily limited to a smaller number of people and perspectives than the evaluation will subsequently consider. Previously undetected agendas may only become clear as data collection and analysis proceeds.

Changes in the climate surrounding the interprofessional education may provide the drivers for new agendas that were not present when the evaluation was designed. The emergence of new or previously undetected agendas should trigger a review of the evaluation plan. Sometimes adjustments are warranted. On other occasions the evaluation can proceed as planned, but with greater sensitivity to the complexity of the local context.

Evaluation is centred on making thoughtful judgements and promoting improvement. It is almost inevitable that there will be people who feel threatened by this process. They may feel moved to attempt a little sabotage: perhaps withholding vital information and then querying its exclusion in your reports; perhaps reacting just slowly enough to put pressure on the evaluation timetable, whilst still being seen to cooperate; losing promised artefacts and forgetting other commitments. Later on, they may persistently question the accuracy and completeness of the evaluation findings. These emergent agendas present threats to the completion and credibility of the evaluation. You need to be vigilant about this and be prepared to review and replan, and, where possible, allay the fears that are generating the resistances.

Evaluators should not expect to be popular with all stakeholders or particular stakeholders at particular times. Nevertheless, evaluators should strive to be sensitive to people's feelings, while remaining fair to all stakeholder groups and rigorous in conducting the evaluation. It is also important to examine the nature and causes of any resistances. Those involved may have valid and important concerns that the evaluation team should incorporate in the evaluation plan and findings.

The effect of the evaluation

It is almost impossible to evaluate interprofessional education without the evaluation itself affecting the development, delivery and participants' assessments of that interprofessional education. Whether this is a strength or a problem depends largely on the evaluation objectives and design. Action-research studies and developmental evaluations are meant to identify areas that would benefit from change and also support the change process. Efficacy studies would try to minimise the impact of the evaluation during the period of data collection.

The 'Hawthorne effect' (Mayo, 1952) is a term used to describe a phenomenon where the behaviour of participants in situations under evaluation changes in response to the presence of the evaluation and the inferred special interest in participants' views and actions. This normally improves outcomes. This effect has also been termed 'researcher reactivity'. Developmental evaluations often seek to generate and harness a Hawthorne effect. Nevertheless, it has been argued that where an evaluator remains involved with participants for longer periods, for example when undertaking observations of learners on an interprofessional course for a period of months, altered behaviour tends to revert back to normal behaviour (Becker, 1970).

Assessing the detailed impact of a Hawthorne effect is complex. At minimum, evaluators need to acknowledge its likely presence in their evaluation.

The position and influence of the evaluator

The methodology and methods you select will result in different forms of influence on your evaluation. Try to remain aware of this so that you can acknowledge the impacts on the evaluation design, data analysis and interpretation, trying to make these transparent in evaluation reports. This will help stakeholders to interpret the evaluation accurately. For example, earlier in this chapter we discussed the relative merits of insider and outsider evaluation. This choice will flavour the entire evaluation so it is important to examine and record the likely impacts.

In deductive, hypothesis-testing studies the main evaluator influence is in the framing of the evaluation questions, and in the identification of contexts or populations to be studied. In inductive, illuminating or hypothesis-generating studies the evaluators collect data through some form of purposive sampling and become 'immersed' in the data to produce a synthesising interpretation of the data set. Thus, the evaluators can be regarded as the main 'interpretative instrument'.

In both deductive and inductive evaluations (and many evaluations have both deductive and inductive aspects) the evaluators influence the boundaries within which the study is conducted, the evaluation design, data collection methods and the approach to data analysis. Even where action researchers work collaboratively with participants through cycles of research, action and evaluation, the evaluation team's underlying philosophies and understanding of the action research context will shape their guidance and, therefore, processes and outcomes.

Statistical and practical significance

Statistical and practical significance are not necessarily the same thing. Although statistical significance is only relevant to evaluation designs that permit some form of quantification, the idea of practical significance is important to qualitative studies too. Thinking and writing about the significance of evaluation findings is an important strand, along with clear communication, in ensuring that your evaluation proves useful to stakeholders.

Some evaluation data sets will include measures of change or correlation that can be tested for statistical significance, for example improved scores on tests of knowledge. These might relate to the content of the interprofessional education (for example effective teamwork in relation to child protection, diabetes, rehabilitation, care for the homeless, ethical decision making, etc.). Other measures that can be tested for statistical significance and might be associated with interprofessional education include responses to attitude surveys at two or more time points, recruitment to particular courses or practice areas, numbers of cancelled operations, the incidence of deviations from integrated care pathways (see Glossary), infection rates, bed-days per patient, readmission rates, immunisation rates, numbers of reported 'near misses' or critical incidents, numbers and categories of complaints, adverse drug reaction reports, and so on. Below is a selection of studies, drawn from our systematic review (Barr *et al.*, 2005), which have produced statistically significant results following an interprofessional education initiative:

- Enhanced confidence to work as an interprofessional team (Schreiber *et al.*, 2002)
- Improvements in the administration of antibiotics (Clemmer *et al.*, 1999)
- Reduction in clinical error rates (Morey *et al.*, 2002)
- Increased screening rates for chlamydia among adolescents (Shafer *et al.*, 2002)
- Decreases in infection rates for neonatal patients (Horbar *et al.*, 2001)

It is very satisfying to be able to report parametric or non-parametric statistical tests that show statistical significance, but the question still arises: does this change have any practical significance? For example, if there is a statistically significant change in the knowledge of participants in an interprofessional educational initiative will this have any impact on the care clients receive or its cost effectiveness? While increasing knowledge might be a necessary precursor to changing practice it is not usually sufficient: cultural and organisational barriers can prevent the improved knowledge being applied. On the other hand, some changes detected by an evaluation may not reach the level of statistical significance because the sample being tested is too small, but the changes may be felt by stakeholders to have practical significance. This may warrant further investigation and, in the interim, a carefully balanced report that draws attention to the phenomenon and its perceived practical significance without making unwarranted statistical claims.

Correlation and causation

Correlation and causation are often confused so we will say a little about them here. Aspects of the interprofessional education that move in step with one another are correlated, for example the perceived relevance of the course content to immediate problem-solving needs is likely to be correlated with satisfaction ratings on feedback questionnaires. There is positive correlation if one measure increases with the other. There is negative correlation if an increase in one measure is associated with a decrease in the other. The size of the correlation (always in the interval 0–1) depends on the degree to which a change in one variable predicts the change that will be observed in the other variable. The size of a correlation coefficient can be tested for statistical significance. However, the presence of correlation between variables, even strong statistically significant correlation, does not imply causation. The two variables may simply both be moving in step with another factor, or the correlation may have just been a coincidence. Even when causation is present, great care has to be taken to establish and communicate its direction: did A cause B, or B cause A?

Conclusion

Following the fundamental decisions (discussed in Chapter nine) about the audience for an evaluation, its purposes and questions, its methodology and design, in this chapter we turned to a web of further issues to be addressed as your evaluation plan develops. We characterised evaluation as an exchange of expertise and knowledge among stakeholders and evaluators: an exchange conducted with guidance from governance and ethics procedures and codes. After securing sufficient preliminary understanding of the evaluation context and negotiating access to people, places and records, a formal evaluation plan will be drawn up to guide the conduct of the evaluation and permit scrutiny by others. The evaluation plan has to be subject to regular review to respond to early findings and changes in the local context. We discussed the effect that an evaluation will have on the interprofessional initiative that is being studied; and the influence of evaluators and their methodological choices on the findings of an evaluation. We also drew attention to the difference between statistical and practical significance, and the non-equivalence of correlation and causation. The next chapter will focus on the resources that will be needed to conduct a successful evaluation of interprofessional education.

Key points

- Evaluation can be regarded as an exchange of perspectives and expertise among evaluators and stakeholders in the interprofessional education. All parties contribute to the evaluation and it can be constructed so that all parties gain from it.

- Evaluations of interprofessional education must be conducted ethically and with due regard for the governance procedures operating in different contexts.
- Plan carefully, but still expect change to be forced upon the evaluation and be prepared for early findings to suggest changes to the remainder of the evaluation.
- Be mindful of the effect of the evaluation on its environment, and the influence of the evaluators.
- Statistical and practical significance are not necessarily the same thing: likewise correlation and causation.

Further reading

Freeth, D., Hammick, M., Barr, H., Koppel, I. & Reeves, S. (2002) *A Critical Review of Evaluations of Interprofessional Education*. LTSN HS&P, London. Available online at http://www.health.ltsn.ac.uk/publications/occasionalpaper/(accessed 5 July 2004).

Gorard, S. (2001) *Quantitative Methods in Educational Research: the Role of Numbers Made Easy*. Continuum, London.

Øvretveit, J. (1998) *Evaluating Health Initiatives: an Introduction to Evaluation of Health Treatments, Services, Policies and Organisational Initiatives*. Open University Press, Buckingham.

Pawson, R. & Tilly N. (1997) *Realistic Evaluation*. Sage, London.

Robson, C. (2002) *Real World Research: a Resource for Social Scientists and Practitioner Researchers*. 2nd edn. Blackwell Publishing, Oxford.

See also further reading in previous chapter.

11 Resources for Evaluations

A range of resources will be required to conduct your evaluation. Your evaluation plan should include securing these in adequate supply and in a timely fashion. The most important resources are time, money, expertise, access and equipment (including software and evaluation instruments). We discussed access in the previous chapter and will now turn to the other types of evaluation resource.

Time and money

Time and money are so closely intertwined that we will discuss them together. It is important to develop a realistic evaluation plan, well matched to the time and money available, and, where necessary, limiting the number of questions addressed and the amount of data collected. Rushed planning, mis-timed data collection, scant analysis, cursory dissemination and superficial action planning are all risks posed by an inadequately resourced evaluation. These deficiencies also represent wasted time and money in a poorly executed evaluation.

The largest cost within an evaluation of interprofessional education will be the evaluators' time (regardless of whether there is explicit funding of this resource). Examples of other costs are shown in Box 11.1.

Developing a well-elaborated list of evaluation tasks and fitting these into a clear timetable helps to ensure that adequate time and money are allocated to each phase of the evaluation. The timetable will need to take account of the ebb and flow of the delivery of the interprofessional education. For example, if a number of parallel groups of learners simultaneously undertake interprofessional education in contrasting settings you may find yourself wanting to conduct observations or focus group interviews in several places at once. This necessitates resource-aware and methodologically informed decisions about how and where to collect data and the human resources required at each phase of the evaluation. It may focus attention on the possible use of naturally occurring data (for example attendance records, assessment data, audit data), the availability of interested people in the locality who might assist with data collection, the short-term use of freelance data collectors, less labour-intensive ways of gathering data, and so on.

The timing and duration of an evaluation also depends on the type of questions that are being asked and the intended uses for the evaluation findings. For example, formative evaluation for the next cycle of delivery necessarily operates

Box 11.1   Possible costs associated with educational evaluations.

- Purchasing specific expertise, such as advice from a statistician or transcribing of recorded interviews.
- Fees for the use of specialised data collection instruments.
- Purchase or hire of evaluation equipment (e.g. mini-disk recording machines, high quality microphones) or data management and analysis software.
- Travel costs to data collection sites and specialist libraries, or for evaluation steering group members to attend meetings.
- Dissemination costs (e.g. printing, the development of a project website, presenting the evaluation at professional meetings).
- Overheads to the organisation hosting the evaluation (for providing office space, computers, financial and human resources management, and basic consumables such as photocopying, telephones and stationery).

to a schedule that is dictated by review, approval and delivery timetables. This almost certainly means swift working and limited scope for negotiation of the evaluation timetable. The advantage of rapid cycles of development is that if aspects of the evaluation have to be cut to meet deadlines another cycle will arrive shortly and permit later implementation of the remainder of the evaluation plan that was agreed with stakeholders. Naturally, this would be subject to renegotiation in the light of findings from the first cycle. In contrast, long-term follow-up studies operate at a rather different pace, but their careful planning and tight execution is very important. There may be no natural second chances to remedy deficiencies in data collection.

An evaluation timetable should be scrutinised for points at which delays or other problems might be predicted to occur. It is useful to plan from the outset strategies for minimising the effects of predictable delays or over-runs. This will leave you better placed to cope with genuinely unforeseeable problems. It is all too easy to underestimate the amount of time required to develop an adequate initial understanding of the local and wider context; to negotiate the scope of the evaluation and hone evaluation questions; select an appropriate methodology and appropriate methods; locate or develop and pilot evaluation instruments; secure ethical approval; collect and sort data; analyse and interpret; write up and present findings in a variety of styles to meet the needs of a variety of stakeholders; and finally, contribute in whatever ways you can to ensuring that learning from the evaluation is used to inform subsequent developments. Evaluation timetables need to schedule time for thinking and preparing, time (and sufficient people) for each of the tasks associated with gathering and interpreting data, and time for writing reports and presentations that will inform subsequent developments.

Resources for formative evaluation of interprofessional education initiatives should be included in the basic costing of each initiative. Evaluations that are likely to yield generalisable findings may also be funded via competitive application to research and development grant programmes. Your local research development office should be able to provide advice on grant givers and alerting services for calls for applications.

Expertise

Your expertise as an educational evaluator will determine the type of evaluation design that you favour and can execute competently. For example, if you lack confidence with statistical analysis you may, however unwittingly, avoid evaluation designs that would necessitate this activity. This can lead to getting stuck in a rut or bending evaluation questions to fit your expertise rather than the needs of stakeholders. Avoidance due to limited expertise is quite different from the defensible position of adopting an informed epistemological stance that, for example, a quantitative, inferential or modelling approach is not suitable for the particular context or stakeholder needs. To guard against avoidance, errors or tunnel vision due to limited expertise it may be helpful to assemble an evaluation team with varying levels and fields of evaluation expertise.

The evaluation team does not have to supply all the expertise required for an evaluation; short-term help can be purchased. For example, you might seek the advice of a statistician; employ a consultant to design a web-based questionnaire, or use a data entry or data transcription service. Another way to broaden the expertise available to an evaluation is to assemble a steering group or panel of critical friends. These people can review evaluation plans, progress and emergent analyses, providing constructive criticism and suggesting alternative perspectives.

Equipment and software

Equipment and software, from the very basic to highly specialist, is available to assist the work at different stages of your evaluation. Hire or purchase costs for the three broad categories (data collection, data analysis and writing up) discussed below, need to be included in your evaluation proposal. First, it is important to have access to secure storage for data and portable equipment. Evaluation data artefacts quickly mount up so ask for a large lockable cupboard.

If you are intending to collect interviews or observations, you should consider obtaining recording equipment. While you can record these data manually in the form of notes, greater accuracy and richness can be obtained by using electronic recorders (audiotape, minidisk or, less commonly, videotape). However, bear in mind that the richer data will take longer to analyse and this may create a sense of overload. The specification of recording equipment needs to be sufficiently high to obtain clear recordings for analysis. It is very upsetting to lose data due to intermittent or inaudible recording, both for evaluators and for those who took the time and trouble to contribute data. Minidisk recorders are popular because the digital recordings they make are significantly clearer than those made on audiotapes. The microphones you select are particularly important and should be well suited to the purposes and environmental conditions of use. Suppliers usually offer a range of options and informed advice. Always practise using recording equipment or other evaluation equipment before you find yourself using it in a situation that can never be replicated. And be sure to carry spare batteries if the equipment you are using depends on these for its power source.

If you plan to transcribe your own audio or video materials it would be wise to investigate transcribing machines that help to make this time consuming (and often tedious) task swifter and more accurate. Transcribing machines enable easy pausing, replaying of short sections and even the slowing of playback whilst deciphering particularly difficult passages. Voice recognition software can assist with the transcribing process if you have high quality recordings, but a human ear will be needed for recordings with significant levels of background noise or feedback, and moments when more than one person is talking. With the aid of specialist software, digital recordings can be uploaded directly to your computer in preparation for data analysis. However, storing audio and video data is resource hungry and you may need to upgrade the memory capacity of your computer. Careful checking of any computer-generated transcripts will be needed to ensure accuracy.

Other specialist software that you might consider includes packages that help to generate questionnaire layouts for paper-based or web-based completion. Well-designed electronic questionnaires present only those questions that are relevant in the light of earlier answers. They may also generate alerts when a respondent skips a question. Answers to electronic questionnaires can be automatically collated and stored in a format that can be accessed by specialist data analysis software.

A wide range of specialist data analysis software is available to support quantitative and qualitative data analysis, although the responsibility for interpretation will remain with the evaluation team. Software should facilitate the linking and comparison of multiple documents. Diagrams (including representations of the coding structure), graphs and tables can be produced for export into reports and presentations. Bibliographic software packages provide a helpful database to store and retrieve details of publications that you read throughout the life of your evaluation.

The choice of evaluation software is very wide so do seek advice and explore demonstration versions of any packages you plan to purchase. Demonstration versions are often freely available from the Internet. Informal networks of peers are useful sources of advice or there may be a software advisory team in your organisation.

Laptop or handheld computers may be important for evaluators who will work away from their main office base for significant periods. Whether a laptop could obviate the need for a desktop PC at the main evaluation base depends upon the specification of the laptop and the arrangements for 'docking' to any networked resources.

Evaluation instruments

Evaluation instruments include questionnaires, observation checklists, interview prompts and data extraction sheets for use with naturally occurring records. Data collection should be fit for purpose and cost effective; good instruments help to achieve this. You may need to develop some evaluation instruments that meet the unique requirements of your evaluation, but, where possible, think about using pre-validated instruments. This will save time and resources that would otherwise be necessary for piloting and validating bespoke instruments. Using pre-tested or standardised evaluation instruments will also increase the scope for comparison of your evaluation findings with those from other contexts.

Well designed data collection instruments will help you to format data in ways that make analysis and checking easy. If you do need to design your own instrument remember to think about how you will want to use and analyse the information it generates. Piloting is also essential because people interpret words, instructions and questions in so many different ways. We will return to piloting in the next chapter, but first a few words about piloted and refined data collection instruments that could be applied to evaluations of interprofessional education.

Research tools developed specifically for the evaluation of interprofessional education include: the Interdisciplinary Education Perception Scale (IEPS, Box 11.2), the Interprofessional Attitudes Questionnaire (IAQ, Box 11.3), the increasingly widely used Readiness for Interprofessional Learning Scale (RIPLS, Box 11.4) and the more recently developed Role Perception Questionnaire (RPQ, Box 11.5).

Box 11.2   The Interdisciplinary Education Perception Scale.

The 18-item IEPS was developed by Luecht *et al.* (1990) in the USA as a pre-test and post-test tool to measure changes in learners' attitudes resulting from a practice-based interprofessional education course. IEPS is constructed around the four factors: professional competence and autonomy, perceived need for collaboration, perceptions of actual collaboration and attitudes towards the contributions of other professions. Use of the IEPS by Hayward *et al.* (1996) revealed that the scale was helpful in identifying changes in health care students' attitudes towards one another following their involvement in a practice-based interprofessional course.

Box 11.3   Interprofessional Attitudes Questionnaire.

The IAQ was developed in the UK by Carpenter (1995a, b) and Carpenter & Hewstone (1996) for their evaluations of interprofessional courses for medical and nursing students, and medical and social work students. It measures participants' attitudes towards other professional groups sharing an interprofessional course. Designed as a pre- and post-test tool, the IAQ contains scales allowing participants to rate: their own profession (to assess auto-stereotypes); other professions on the course (to assess hetero-stereotypes); their own profession as seen by others (to assess perceived auto-stereotypes). Use of the IAQ in a number of interprofessional education evaluations (e.g. Barnes *et al.*, 2000; Hind *et al.*, 2003) has provided illuminating data in relation to participants' attitudes to one another.

Box 11.4   Readiness for Interprofessional Learning Scale.

The RIPLS was developed in the UK by Parsell & Bligh (1999) to measure student attitudes to interprofessional learning. The original scale consists of 19 statements arranged in three subscales (teamwork and collaboration, professional identity and roles and responsibilities). Large-scale validation of the scale is ongoing, drawing data from the UK and other countries. It has been lengthened to include a fourth subscale. Use of the RIPLS by, for example, Horsburgh *et al.* (2001), Hind *et al.* (2003), Morison *et al.* (2003) has revealed this tool to be a useful pre-initiative measure of student attitudes to interprofessional education.

Box 11.5   Role Perception Questionnaire.

Mackay (2004) describes the development and validation of two versions of a Role perception questionnaire. First, the 20-item generic role perception questionnaire (GRPQ), based on personal constructs elicited from senior students, in England, from eight professions (midwifery, nursing, occupational therapy, physiotherapy, podiatry, prosthetics and orthotics, radiography and social work). Second, a 31-item nursing role perception questionnaire (NRPQ) with seven factors. Work is ongoing to produce other profession-specific RPQs and to identify normative values. These promise to be useful, rigorously constructed additions to the range of resources available for evaluating interprofessional education.

The teamwork literature also offers a large number of instruments, some of which may well be helpful where interprofessional education aims to improve teamwork. A small selection of well validated teamwork instruments that have proved useful in health or social care settings is presented below (Boxes 11.6–11.9). A more comprehensive description and critique of teamwork

---

Box 11.6   Team Climate Inventory.

Developed in the UK for primary care teams, the Team Climate Inventory (Anderson & West, 1994, 1998) is a set of four separate but interrelated scales designed to measure different aspects of a team's collaborative processes: team objectives, team participation, quality and support for innovation. Use of this inventory (e.g. Williams & Laungani 1999; Gibbon *et al.*, 2002) has revealed that it is a helpful tool in measuring the nature of team processes in a number of health care and management teams. The Team climate inventory might offer a useful pre-course/post-course instrument for evaluating the impact of interprofessional education on the nature and quality of teamwork within an established health/social care team.

Box 11.7   Team Effectiveness Questionnaire.

The Team Effectiveness Questionnaire, developed and subsequently used in UK-based primary care by Poulton & West (1993, 1994, 1999) is a 25-item instrument designed to measure how effective a team is in relation to four dimensions of effectiveness: teamwork, organisational efficiency, health care practices and patient-centred care. The Team effectiveness questionnaire might be a helpful tool for assessing the impact of interprofessional education on the quality and effectiveness of teamwork within an established health/social care team.

Box 11.8   The System for Multiple Level Observations of Groups.

The SYMLOG (System for Multiple Level Observation of Groups), developed in the USA by Bales & Cohen (1979) is a 26-item rating scale used to measure individual group members' perceptions of other members based on three dimensions: prominence (how active, dominant and assertive); sociability (e.g. warmth, friendliness); and task orientation (e.g. rationality towards tasks and task-focused). Farrell *et al.* (2001b) usefully employed SYMLOG in their evaluation of informal roles in health care teams, including assessing how individual informal roles within teams evolved over time. SYMLOG was also used by Cashman (2004).

Box 11.9 Interaction Process Analysis Instrument.

Bales' (1976) Interaction process analysis instrument was devised in the USA to categorise and understand the socio-emotional and task-oriented nature of interaction within groups or teams. The observation of interaction within a group is based on assigning behaviour to the following categories: solidarity/ antagonism; displaying/releasing tension; agreeing/disagreeing; giving/ asking for suggestions; giving/asking for opinions and giving/asking for orientation. In recording interaction between group members within these categories, Bales' tool aims to understand the issues and process around communication, control and decision making. The Interaction process analysis tool might provide a helpful insight into the nature of interactions that occur during an interprofessional course.

---

scales can be found in Heinemann & Zeiss (2002). Whilst not an evaluation instrument, we will be discussing our classification of the outcomes of interprofessional education at the end of Chapter twelve (see also Table 2.1). This classification can be a useful resource when planning an evaluation, securing preliminary understanding of the multifaceted nature of interprofessional education and its evaluation, or when organising data and interpretations from your evaluation.

It is important to appreciate that evaluation instruments that have undergone piloting and validation to prove their worth in particular contexts and to establish their psychometric properties are coherent wholes meant for the contexts in which they were validated. First, they may not be as valid or reliable in your evaluation context, so care and professional judgement will be required. Second, it is not possible to pick only certain questions from within a scale, or to change wording without destroying the prior validation that might have been the justification for choosing that evaluation instrument. Of course, you will need to change words that have no resonance or, worse, have different meanings in your context. Just remember that the psychometric properties of the scale may change and that simple comparisons need to become more sophisticated comparisons with other evaluations, using the instrument in other contexts (with or without their own minor modifications).

If questionnaires or interviews are to be administered by several members of the evaluation team, or this data collection is to be subcontracted to temporary field workers, comprehensive training in the use of the evaluation instruments becomes particularly important. You will want to know that everyone is using the instruments as consistently as possible and in harmony with the evaluation plan.

Conclusion

When planning an evaluation it is all too easy to underestimate the amount of time required to develop an adequate initial understanding of the local and wider context; to negotiate the scope of the evaluation and hone evaluation questions; select an appropriate methodology and appropriate methods; locate or develop and pilot evaluation instruments (for example questionnaires, interview schedules); secure ethical approval; collect and sort data; analyse and interpret; write up and present findings in a variety of styles to meet the needs of a variety of stakeholders; and finally, contribute in whatever ways you can to ensuring that learning from the evaluation is used to inform subsequent developments. Developing a well elaborated list of evaluation tasks helps to ensure that adequate time and money are allocated to each phase of the evaluation. The timetable will need to take account of the ebb and flow of the delivery of the interprofessional education.

Evaluation plans need to be matched to the time, expertise and other resources that are available. A wide range of specialist equipment and software is available to assist evaluators, and an increasing range of evaluation instruments that are suitable for examining different facets of interprofessional education.

Key points

- Recognise the range of resources required for evaluation and make considered choices. Include these in the evaluation plan.
- Schedule time for thinking and preparing, time (and sufficient people) for each of the tasks associated with gathering and interpreting data, and time for reports and presentations that will inform subsequent developments.
- Develop a well elaborated list of evaluation tasks to help ensure that adequate resources are allocated to each phase of the evaluation.
- Take account of the ebb and flow of the delivery of the interprofessional education.
- Evaluator(s) time is the largest evaluation cost. See Box 11.1 for examples of other costs.
- Data collection should be fit for purpose and cost effective; good instruments help to achieve this.
- Train the team of data collectors and coders so that they work as consistently as possible and in harmony with the evaluation plan.

Further reading

Denscombe, M. (2003) *The Good Research Guide: for Small-scale Research Projects*. Open University Press, Buckingham.

Fink, A. (2002) (ed) *The Survey Kit* Vol. 1. Sage, London.

Oppenheim, A. (1999) *Questionnaire Design, Interviewing and Attitudes Measurement*. Pinter, London.

12 Conducting Evaluations

Introduction

In this chapter we will focus on issues that arise as evaluations of interprofessional education get underway, including: the ongoing quest for clarity, facets of trust and credibility, pilot studies and baseline data collection, then ongoing data management and analysis. Finally, we will return to our classification of the outcomes of interprofessional education, continuing the discussion we began in Chapter two.

Striving for clarity

In an ideal world the evaluation of interprofessional education would not proceed without all stakeholders achieving clarity on:

- The meaning of interprofessional education
- The intended nature and objectives of the particular interprofessional education initiative under evaluation
- The boundaries of the interprofessional education and the boundaries of the evaluation
- The purpose and methodological approach of the evaluation
- The roles and responsibilities of different people, groups and organisations

In reality, conceptions of interprofessional education and its evaluation vary. Although efforts should be made to explicate and align people's conceptions and aspirations, it is unlikely that everyone concerned with an initiative will view things the same way. The boundaries between an initiative and its environment may be blurred, making it harder to delimit the evaluation. Of course, evaluators should and do strive for the highest levels of clarity possible, paying particular attention to areas that are critical to the validity and credibility of the evaluation. But ultimately it is necessary to move forward pragmatically, tolerating a certain level of ambiguity. Nevertheless, the evaluation process and evaluation reports can (and should aspire to) contribute to enhancing clarity of thought and understanding.

Trust and credibility

Evaluations of interprofessional education will raise questions of trustworthiness and credibility in a variety of ways. First, we will look at human interaction and ethical practice, and then turn to methodological conceptions of trustworthiness and credibility.

Human interaction and ethical practice

Those that commission and facilitate the evaluation will want to feel confident that the evaluation team is credible and has a credible evaluation plan. This is established in a variety of ways, but particularly through written and verbal interactions, including: negotiating the form and scope of the evaluation, a formal evaluation proposal, interactions during data collection, discussion of preliminary findings and interactions during the period in which the evaluation team helps to promote informed development.

Aspects of trust and credibility can be scrutinised in the evaluation plan. For example:

- Is there appropriate linkage between the evaluation questions, methodology, and methods of data collection and analysis?
- Are plans for sampling (random, stratified, systematic, cluster, theoretical, purposive, convenience, snowball, etc.)[1] appropriate for the evaluation methodology and adequately justified?
- Are any ethical concerns raised by the evaluation design adequately addressed?

The evaluation team may be given access to documents of commercial value that are not in the public domain. Evaluators will need to check carefully which aspects of these documents may be referenced in any report, and which details may or may not be revealed within and outside the organisation during data collection. For example, access to minutes for one organisation participating in the interprofessional education may reveal their impending withdrawal from the project. You will need to find out when their partner organisations will be informed of this and take care not to inadvertently 'leak' the news. In situations such as this it is important to be alert to attempts to use the evaluation team as an unofficial conduit for important information.

Normally, evaluators seek to provide the highest feasible degree of confidentiality and anonymity for evaluation participants; particularly for relatively power-

[1] We will not discuss sampling in any detail within this chapter but we have provided some brief notes within the Glossary. A wide variety of evaluation and research methods texts available to inform sampling decisions including: Rossi *et al.* (1985), Henry (1990), Cohen *et al.* (2000), Oppenheim (2000), Mason (2002), Patton (2002).

less participants such as students or junior members of staff, or for isolated participants such as the single occupant of a key role. To a great extent this can be achieved by aggregating data and by limiting the identifying features within quotations. For particularly sensitive material the evaluators might take active steps to disguise the identity of people or places, but this should not be undertaken lightly because it raises a number of questions. Is this action justifiable? Is it likely to successfully protect the source? Will this action distort the evaluation messages?

Realistically, certain roles and individuals will be identifiable from the evaluation data they contribute, particularly to members of their own organisation. Providing key informants with draft copies of pertinent sections from evaluation reports can avert unnecessary distress. Time for checking with key informants therefore needs to be factored into the reporting schedule.

The evaluation team needs clear guidance for circumstances in which confidentiality will be broken in order to prevent more serious harm, and the mechanisms for doing this. If the evaluators are health or social care professionals their professions' codes of conduct may adequately provide the necessary framework. Social scientists working in these contexts would probably look towards the codes of conduct developed by their discipline (in the UK this might include the British Educational Research Association: www.bera.ac.uk, the British Psychological Society: bps.org.uk, the British Sociological Association: www.britsoc.co.uk, etc.) in addition to codes developed by the organisations that employ evaluators (universities, health care providers, social services providers, etc.). It is very rare for evaluators to have to set aside the evaluation task and take action to prevent harm, but it is important to realise that the process of evaluation has the potential to stumble across evidence of fraud, negligence or abuse.

Methodological conceptions of trustworthiness and credibility

In addition to the human interaction and ethical practice aspects of trust and credibility, evaluators will be mindful of the conceptions of trustworthiness and credibility that apply to the evaluation methodology they have chosen. For example, for an evaluation design based on quantitative measurement, scientific conceptions of reliability, validity, replication and generalisability will be relevant. The main questions to ask will include:

- Did we actually measure what we set out to measure?
- Is this what we should have been measuring?
- If we measured again would we get the same answers?
- Did we measure sufficient examples, items or instances from among all that might have been measured?
- Was the sampling appropriate for its purpose?
- What was our response rate and loss to follow-up (attrition), and the implications of these?

- Did we take steps to eliminate as many sources of bias as possible and to estimate the effect of those aspects of bias that remained?
- Were we clear about the type of measure obtained (nominal, ordinal, interval or ratio)?
- Did we choose appropriate tests, apply them correctly and make evidenced inferences?
- Have we indicated levels of confidence that can be attached to our results and inferences?

For an evaluation design based on a qualitative approach, conceptions of trust-worthiness, plausibility, credibility, dependability, auditability, confirmability, authenticity, voice and reflexivity are added to (or for some people replace) those of reliability and validity. Important questions include:

- Have the influences of the evaluation and evaluators been adequately considered?
- Did we pay sufficient attention to the opportunities for bias to enter this study and means for minimising its adverse consequences?
- What guided our sampling and how did this affect what we found?
- Did this evaluation suffer from significant attrition of participants or contexts?
- How should such attrition be interpreted and what caveats should be placed on interpretations from the resultant diminished data set?
- Have emergent theories or hypotheses been tested by negative case analysis or some other means?
- Have descriptions and interpretations been subject to member checking or an equivalent process?
- What types of triangulation were possible and how many of these did we use?
- What did triangulation tell us?

Many of the concepts highlighted in preceding paragraphs are multifaceted, for example validity (internal, external, face, construct, content, predictive, ecological, etc.) and triangulation (theoretical, methodological, investigator, time, space, etc.). We do not have space in this chapter to consider each in detail but there is a wide range of evaluation texts and research methods texts that provide more detailed discussion, for example, Cohen *et al.* (2000), Oppenheim (2000) and Mason (2002) and the texts in the suggested further reading at the end of Chapters nine to twelve. We have also included some brief notes in the Glossary.

Attention to bias

Attention to bias is necessary within both qualitative and quantitative evaluation approaches. Bias may be thought of as over- or underestimating the size or influence of a factor within the evaluation setting, or as over- or underestimating the importance of some aspect of your evaluation.

In quantitative studies bias may occur at the sampling stage. Particular groups or items can be inadvertently over- or under-sampled. This is different to deliberate over-sampling of sparse or hard to reach groups in order to ensure adequate participation; a feature that would be built into subsequent analyses and interpretations. Later in the evaluation response bias may emerge. This means certain groups are more likely to contribute to the evaluation than others, giving their views disproportionate weight. Attrition from the study may also introduce bias. For example, in controlled trials it is more common to suffer attrition in the control group than in initiative groups. This spoils the carefully balanced allocation to groups. Quantitative studies may also overemphasise the role of things that are easy to measure and quantify.

Bias in qualitative evaluations is also concerned with sampling decisions, response patterns and attrition. However, more emphasis is placed on the behaviour of fieldworkers and the epistemological positions of those engaged in the design of the evaluation, analysis and interpretation. Evaluators may notice things that confirm their preconceived ideas and overlook discordant evidence. They may empathise more with certain groups or more readily comprehend their perspectives. These then receive undue emphasis in the evaluation findings. There may be over reliance on accessible or key informants. Evaluators may be unaware of important antecedent events and pay insufficient attention to the resonance and usefulness of findings in other contexts. The presence of evaluators may change behaviour in relation to the interprofessional learning. Evaluators may also 'go native' and lose their ability for critical observation and analysis.

Certain types of bias may be linked to particular study designs or ways of collecting data. For example:

- Leading questions, selective attendance to responses, projection of personal views (verbally or through body language), over-identification with interviewees, or misunderstanding what is said are all potential sources of bias introduced by an interviewer.
- Questionnaire and interview respondents may misunderstand what they have been asked, or deliberately mislead the evaluators.
- In the analysis of archived documents or naturally occurring data, bias is introduced with decisions taken by people without an evaluation role, of what is worthy of keeping or recording.
- Maturation affects all long-term studies. Things naturally change over time and it can be difficult to disentangle the effects of the initiative you are evaluating from natural maturation effects or changes precipitated by other factors.

Bias is a facet of our existence in the world. It cannot be eliminated from evaluations, but there are ways of minimising it. Critical reflection on the design and conduct of an evaluation allows recognition of probable sources of bias and action to control its influence. Action might include: choosing appropriate statistical techniques, careful cleaning and cross-checking of data, reporting findings with suitable caveats and being clear about the limitations of the evaluation. Bias will also be reduced by giving attention to any findings that lie 'outwith' the main body of results and to those that contrast with the majority. This may mean that your evaluation identifies mixed or neutral results, and those that are negative as well as positive. Reporting all of these with sensitivity is part of your duty as an evaluator as we discuss in Chapter thirteen.

Other ways of reducing bias are the use of reflexivity, triangulation, diligently following up non-respondents, obtaining feedback on emergent findings, encouraging critical debate and ensuring that interpretations and recommendations are well warranted by the empirical data. It is worth stressing that evaluations of all types largely find aspects of what they plan to look for: the unanticipated may not be adequately captured or analysed. Drawing expertise from a group with contrasting orientations helps to minimise this problem.

Pilot studies and baseline data collection

Evaluation designs and instruments that you develop will need to be piloted: that is, tried out on a smaller scale than the fully-planned evaluation in order to highlight possible problems and risks. These might include difficulty in identifying or contacting people who should be asked to contribute to the evaluation, poor performance of available equipment (for example microphones) in some of the environments where they will be used, hitherto undocumented changes to the interprofessional education under evaluation, ambiguity in evaluation documents (for example questionnaires, information sheets for participants), insufficient response categories in structured questionnaires, time or timing problems (for example the interview prompts list is too long, choosing/receiving poor slots for data collection).[2]

Piloting and validation occurs at different levels of complexity, appropriate to the purpose of the evaluation instrument. For example, observation checklists and data extraction sheets primarily need to be usable in naturally occurring contexts by the range of field workers that will be attached to your project. Criteria of acceptability include pragmatic questions such as: Are they too bulky to handle or too cramped for the required data entry? There would also need to be attention to the clarity of instructions so that all trained users would extract similar information, reducing the occurrence of fieldworker bias. There must also be scope to note the unanticipated. The pilot study may reveal a need for additional fieldworker training to improve consistency and attain the desired focus and depth; or a need for modification of the schedule (and consequent re-piloting). Cyclical data collection and analysis will establish whether previously unanticipated facets of

---

[2] Poor data collection slots include times when participants are hungry, tired or anxious to get to their next activity or, in the case of access to documentary data when the annual reconciliation, reporting and archiving process is underway or during other peaks of activity such as departmental moves, new student registrations, new employee inductions, etc.

the evaluated context should become anticipated categories for observation or data extraction and thus, checked in all cases. A pilot study would also address the appropriateness of the anticipated categories in relation to the evaluation questions and the observed context, particularly noting whether the categories appeared to be discrete, unambiguous and exhaustive.

As a second example, the piloting of questionnaires enables feedback on the clarity of instructions, questions and the general layout. The success of branches within the questionnaire can be judged, the completion time checked and commonly misunderstood or uncompleted items can be identified for further development. Provisional coding systems and data entry/analysis plans can be tested. Initial piloting and subsequent cycles of data collection and analysis allow for a documented natural evolution of evaluation instruments. The creation of validated scales that have known psychometric properties is a much more technical matter; see, for example, Oppenheim (2000). It requires substantial resources and a context with a large number of potential participants.

Each data collection method and every methodology raises specific piloting issues and fuller discussions can be found in several of the texts in the suggested further reading sections at the end of Chapters nine to twelve. In essence the same process is at work: trying out instruments or approaches, looking for potential problems and risks and then minimising these before they can threaten the main evaluation.

Assuming that pilot studies precede the main evaluation (although early findings may sometimes lead to the introduction of new or modified elements which will require later piloting) the next stage will be baseline data collection. What baseline data is collected depends on your evaluation questions and the opportunities offered by the evaluation context, but it might include attitude measurement, satisfaction surveys, assessment of relevant skills and knowledge, biographical information, audit data, and so on. It is at this phase that you will know more clearly whether you were successful in gaining sufficient preliminary understanding to develop a sound evaluation plan (see Chapter nine).

If the quality of the prior information you obtained and weighed at the securing preliminary understanding phase was poorer than you realised then the quality of your plans may now be threatened. For example, notionally comparable groups or settings may turn out to have significant differences. This will leave you coping with change during the life of your evaluation (see Chapter ten). Whilst it may not be humanly possible to avoid getting caught out once in a while, energy invested in careful planning and piloting goes a long way towards ensuring that you are not needlessly caught out.

Ongoing data collection, data management and data analysis

Data collection, data management and data analysis are cyclical processes in most evaluations of interprofessional education and certainly overlap in all evaluations. We indicated earlier that we do not have space here to discuss data collection methods in detail, and this is done well in many of the texts identified at the end of Chapters nine to twelve as suggestions for further reading. The important points to draw out in relation to data collection are:

- It should be fit for purpose; that is designed to address the evaluation questions that have been agreed with stakeholders, and capable of providing insights that may act as catalysts for evidence-informed change or expansion.
- Data collection should allow the unanticipated to emerge and be recorded. We tend to find aspects of what we set out to look for, but should not exclude the possibility of something far richer or far more important emerging as the evaluation progresses.
- Data collection should cause as little disruption to the work of the interprofessional education or practice setting as possible, not least because disruptive data collection will change the nature of the situation being evaluated, but also because evaluators must recognise patients and clients, health and social care professionals, tutors and students as busy people for whom our evaluation is not their main purposeful activity or first priority.
- Data collection should also be cost effective. This means that it should not be unnecessarily elaborate (for example if you are only interested in the sound track use an audio recorder rather than a video reorder, it will be much quicker to process). Where suitable naturally occurring data exist (for example audit data) the evaluation should make maximum use of these in preference to new data collection. In addition, an important contribution to cost effectiveness is finding means of knowing when you have collected sufficient information for your evaluation.

Experimental studies and other quantitative approaches may use power calculations and other statistical devices to set data collection targets and sampling frameworks in advance. Qualitative studies are more likely to work towards saturation (continuing until nothing new is being learnt) and purposive or theoretical sampling (see, for example, Chapter seven in Mason, 2002). Both approaches to evaluation are most economically executed if data management proceeds in parallel with data collection.

Data should be processed for analysis as soon as possible after its collection. Audio and video recordings may need to be transcribed and formatted for subsequent analysis, and also made anonymous. Documents will need to be catalogued and indexed, and may contain elements that need to be made anonymous. Data processing needs to be checked for accuracy (for example double coding by separate people, double entry on spreadsheets and other databases, proof reading). You might also return interview transcripts to interviewees for checking and annotation. (This is one form of 'member checking' and contributes to the trustworthiness of your evaluation; see the earlier section on methodological conceptions of trustworthiness and credibility.)

Early processing of data will highlight technical problems that can be fixed for subsequent data collection. It may also highlight 'blind spots' in the original data collection strategy that can be addressed before the period available for data collection expires. Safely stored back-up copies of your data set are essential.

Evaluations that are formulated in terms of saturation and purposive or theoretical sampling require data collection, processing and analysis that proceed in (usually rapid) cycles, otherwise you will not know when to stop, or which type of information to seek out next. However, achieving saturation is beyond the resources of most evaluations and, in any case, a law of diminishing returns sets in before saturation. More information might be useful or illuminating but only marginally so, thus making it difficult to justify spending resources on the extra data collection. Wherever your data collection stops you will need to reflect on how close to saturation you appear to be. This will help readers explain your findings and interpretations.

Data analysis has to be well matched to the evaluation questions and the type of data. There are many specialist texts available to help you. We suggest reading fairly general evaluation or research methods texts to examine a range of possibilities and using these as a springboard to more specialised reading. Other possibilities include seeking the advice of colleagues or membership of on-line discussion groups and searching relevant websites. Some techniques may be best learnt within the social interaction provided by training workshops or through the coaching of experienced users.

Data analysis is not a single process. A thorough initial analysis will lay bare the most obvious features of your data set. Inspection of the initial analysis should generate hypotheses or new questions; these will send you back to the data set (perhaps even back to data collection) for a second sweep of data analysis and interpretation. As this iterative process continues, more nuanced understandings and more sophisticated models emerge. Follow-up work beyond the scope of your current evaluation of interprofessional education may also be signalled and planning can commence in parallel with the completion, dissemination and use of the ongoing evaluation. Sharing and using the findings from your evaluation will be our focus in the next chapter.

Our classification of outcomes of interprofessional education

Finally, we return to the classification of outcomes of interprofessional education that we developed in the course of our systematic reviews of evaluations of interprofessional education. This is displayed in Table 2.1. Our classification, the evolution of which is described in Freeth *et al.* (2002, p. 13–14), extends the classic Kirkpatrick outcomes model which is described at length in Thackwray (1997). It has proved sufficient to guide data extraction and classify outcomes from over 350 evaluations of interprofessional education identified by our systematic reviewing and would be a useful guide for designing or reporting new evaluations of interprofessional education. The classification is not hierarchical in terms of the importance of outcomes but the difficulty of gathering and interpreting evaluation varies across the levels.

Our review work indicates that saturation may have been reached with respect to descriptive studies focused on learners' reactions to interprofessional education (level 1). There were relatively few studies focused on levels 2a and 3. Of the studies focused on levels 4a and 4b, most involved post-qualification learners and the interprofessional education was usually part of a quality improvement initiative. More details of our review methodology and findings can be found in our companion volume Barr *et al.* (2005). Boxes 12.1 to 12.6 provide examples of evaluations focused at various levels within the classification.

Conclusion

Strong, achievable evaluations of interprofessional education begin with hard thinking that results in a clear conception of the journey ahead. Incisive thinking at the planning stage saves time later and yields results that you can be proud of. However, review and consequent replanning are also integral parts of the

---

Box 12.1   An example of an evaluation reporting level 1 outcomes, UK.

Doyle *et al.* (2003) described an evaluation of a short interprofessional workshop designed for mental health care practitioners working in Salford and Manchester. After carrying out a needs assessment with staff, a two-day seminar-based workshop was developed, focusing on the management of clinical risk. The course was delivered to over 200 practitioners working in mental health trusts and social services departments (doctors, nurses and unspecified 'others').

The course was evaluated using questionnaires. Initially, questionnaires were distributed to all participants directly after the course. To understand the longer-term impact a 12-month follow-up questionnaire was sent to a random sample of 100 participants. Initially, 94% of participants rated the course as 'good' or 'excellent'. In particular, participants stated that they enjoyed the interprofessional interaction. Similar views were expressed by the participants who completed a follow-up questionnaire.

The authors concluded that the high levels of satisfaction expressed by the participants indicated that the course provided them with a useful introduction to the management of clinical risk. They went on to note that more advanced workshops or refresher courses were being developed to ensure that practitioners' understanding of these issues could be deepened.

Box 12.2   An example of an evaluation reporting level 2a outcomes.

Gibbon *et al.* (2002) examined the impact on teamwork of introducing an integrated care pathway (ICP) and a new unified system of recording patient notes (PNs) for staff involved in stroke care in the UK. Before the introduction of these new systems, staff were offered a series of interprofessional education sessions designed to help understand how to work together following the implementation of both the ICP and the PN system. Four stroke rehabilitation units took part in the initiative: two introduced the ICP and two introduced the PN system. The authors adopted a before-and-after research design and employed the Team climate inventory (see Box 11.6) to examine whether staff felt these new systems had affected the quality of their teamwork. Staff in three of the units reported only marginal improvements in the perceived quality of teamwork and staff in the fourth unit (implemented PN system) reported deterioration in their views of the quality of teamwork. The authors stated that more management support was required to facilitate change and to demonstrate commitment to the new systems.

---

evaluation process. Evaluation is a complex social interaction, an exchange between people with many different perspectives. The evaluation must generate trust and work with disciplinary differences in conceptions of credibility. The design and orientation of the evaluation strongly influence the smoothness of its execution, the perspectives it elicits and the conclusions it draws. Throughout Chapters nine to twelve we have focused on the processes and decisions involved in translating a sound evaluation plan into a soundly executed evaluation. Data collection, analysis and interpretation were described as cyclical activities. Evaluations were seen as meeting local needs and both informing and being informed by wider debates.

Box 12.3   An example of an evaluation reporting level 2b outcomes.

Farrell *et al.* (2001a) described an evaluation of an interprofessional 'breaking bad news' workshop. Designed to enhance communication skills and understanding of one another's roles, a one-day workshop was offered to practitioners working in a range of paediatric settings. These included accident and emergency, intensive care, general medical and surgical clinical areas. In each workshop, staff discussed a range of patient cases and undertook role-play exercises. Forty-five nurses and doctors participated. To understand the impact of this initiative, staff completed questionnaires directly after their workshop. Findings suggested that the workshops had enhanced the participants' communication skills and improved their knowledge of each other's professional roles.

Box 12.4   An example of an evaluation reporting level 3 outcomes.

Berman *et al.* (2000) reported an evaluation of a series of interprofessional sessions for 19 physicians, physiotherapists, occupational therapists, social workers and psychologists, working in an outpatient rehabilitation clinic for children with disabilities in the USA. Staff members were offered 16 weekly one-hour sessions, which were designed to enhance their ability to collaborate more effectively in practice. The evaluation aimed to investigate the differences in team functioning before and after the delivery of the sessions. Observations of these practitioners' interprofessional team meetings were collected by video and assessed against the Transdisciplinary Team Participation Scale (TTPS), a pre-validated instrument devised to measure participation in a team meeting. Compared with pre-session scores, post-session scores on the TTPS revealed that staff members' participation during their interprofessional meetings had significantly increased. The authors concluded that a series of short interprofessional team-based sessions can improve the team participation, which in turn should mean that information between team members is shared more effectively.

Box 12.5   An example of an evaluation reporting level 4a outcomes.

Lalonde *et al.* (2002) provided a report of their evaluation into the effects of an interprofessional course for health and social care practitioners working in nine sexual health community clinics in the USA. The course aimed to increase practitioners' understanding of HIV/AIDS and enhance their approaches to working together in delivering care to clients. It consisted of a series of interactive workshops, computer-based distance learning and didactic presentations. In total, 598 practitioners from medicine, nursing, dentistry, social work, counselling and outreach work participated. To understand its impact on practice, follow-up telephone interviews were undertaken eight months after the course with 218 purposively selected participants. Most participants (87%) reported improvements in the way the clinics operated. In particular, inter-agency referrals were felt to be better targeted and inter-agency liaison had improved. It was also reported that clinical assessments and treatment plans were better targeted; and the quality of each clinic's documentation was enhanced.

> **Box 12.6**   An example of an evaluation reporting level 4b outcomes.
>
> Morey *et al.* (2002) reported an evaluation of a team-based course for doctors, nurses and technicians working in the emergency departments of nine teaching hospitals in the USA. The course aimed to enhance each team's ability to collaborate in an effective manner, by offering training into the use of the aviation crew resource management model of teamwork. A controlled before and after research design was adopted to assess the effectiveness of the training on interprofessional collaboration. Six of the emergency departments were assigned into the experimental group (to receive the training): the remaining three departments provided the control group. Questionnaire data gathered from the participants and their patients revealed that while patient satisfaction scores remained unchanged across both experimental and control groups, the clinical error rate decreased significantly in the experimental group.

Key points

- Try to obtain a high level of clarity about objectives and boundaries.
- Pay attention to trust, credibility and ethical dilemmas.
- Conduct pilot studies to test new evaluation designs or instruments.
- Collect, process and analyse evaluation data in cycles rather than a single linear sequence, to prevent wastage and to permit the identification of gaps while they might still be rectified.

Further reading

Denzin, N. & Lincoln, Y. (eds) (2000) *Handbook of Qualitative Research*. 2nd edn. Sage, London.

Hart, E. & Bond, M. (1995) *Action Research for Health and Social Care: A Guide to Practice*. Open University Press, Milton Keynes.

Mason, J. (2002) *Qualitative Researching*. 2nd edn. Sage, London.

May, T. (ed.) (2002) *Qualitative Research in Action*. Sage, London.

Silverman, D. (1999) *Doing Qualitative Research: A Practical Handbook*. Sage, London.

See also further reading in Chapters nine to eleven.

13 Using and Sharing Learning from Evaluations

Introduction

Evaluation findings are meant to be used to improve the interprofessional education that was studied and interprofessional education in other contexts; they may also be used to improve the practice of evaluating interprofessional education. For this to happen there is a need for effective communication and discussion about the evaluation process and findings with stakeholders from the local context and the wider professional and interprofessional education communities. This is more than just writing an evaluation report; such documents do not necessarily speak for themselves. The evaluation team's responsibility includes ensuring that effective communication has occurred and identifying discussion opportunities. Sharing and using findings can be central to the evaluation throughout its life; part of the dynamic relationship between policy, practice and research.

In this chapter we discuss the timing of evaluation feedback and the importance of sharing your evaluation findings with local stakeholders and the wider interprofessional education community. We argue for staged feedback that will enable swifter development of the interprofessional education. This allows initial interpretations of the evaluation data to be strengthened by early exposure to critical review from stakeholders. We also comment on the challenges associated with providing timely staged feedback. This is followed by a discussion about tailoring written and oral dissemination for the range of audiences and purposes that your evaluation may serve. Then we turn our attention to the many facets of communicating clearly and, finally, barriers to using your findings. First, though, we focus on aspects of professionalism in writing evaluation reports and academic papers.

Professional matters

Decisions need to be made about authorship of any publication that reports the work of an evaluation team. These include who is to be an author and the order of their names on the report. A named author should have made a substantial intellectual contribution to the research process, to the drafting of the report or paper and have approved the final published version. Some members of the evaluation team will be largely occupied with data collection, synthesis and interpretation, while others will have intermittent and advisory roles. For a particular report or paper one team member may have taken the role of leading the writing up, with others making lesser but clear contributions. The British Sociological Association (2003) and the International Committee of Medical Journal Editors (2003) provide guidance on this (see further reading at the end of the chapter). It is normal practice to include the name and contact details of one author who has agreed to be responsible for correspondence about the document or paper.

The other matter of professionalism concerns dissemination as an ethical duty. Resources will be dedicated to your evaluation of interprofessional education and the reporting process provides an account of the use of those resources. Even more importantly, a wide range of people will take the time to contribute thoughtfully to your evaluation. They deserve to have their contributions recognised and valued. The dissemination process does this and, if well conducted, will leave participants well disposed towards future evaluations. In the same way as we should all try not to spoil places of beauty with litter or careless damage, we owe it to the wider community of evaluators not to spoil goodwill and trust in evaluation settings.

Internal formative evaluation

Internal formative evaluation usually precedes sharing findings more widely. The internal evaluation is primarily aimed at providing stakeholders (for example those in Figure 2.2) with useful information in a timely manner. For example, course tutors will want to know about participants' feedback on the delivery and perceived usefulness of the interprofessional education in time to inform the next cycle of teaching, learning and assessment. Programme developers will want to know about the participant feedback, any assessment results, the impact of the course on tutors and its impact on the infrastructure services of the participating organisations. Questions they may have include:

- Did the interprofessional education generate an unanticipated surge in library and information services requests?
- Was it more complicated to register and track participants from a variety of professions?
- How did the logistics of getting people together work?
- What was the impact of interprofessional groups of learners on the service areas that hosted them, and also on service users?

Stakeholders who provided resources to support the interprofessional education will want to know how those resources were used, how effective this appeared to be, and what the projected resource implications are as the initiative develops.

Information from the evaluation needs to be useful. Usefulness has several facets, including the timing, focus and style of reports. We say a few words about timing here and return to focus and style later when considering audience and purpose.

Timeliness and staged feedback

Evaluation reports to stakeholders about the ongoing development of the inter-professional education need, so far as is possible, to reach them before decisions on the next cycle of delivery are due. This may not always be possible because the lead times for changes to certain accredited or approved programmes can some-times be several months (Chapter eight). In these situations your evaluation may be informing the next-but-one cycle of delivery.

Reporting to stakeholders as swiftly as possible and linked to their schedule of resource allocation and curriculum development meetings is often a challenge. The schedules may be fixed in relation to wider organisational needs, without paying much attention to the feasibility of having appropriate evaluation infor-mation available to meet that timetable. The pressure to report quickly can militate against producing a well balanced and comprehensive account. Some-times this leads to misconceptions that need to be addressed at a later date, but the alternative may be a better account that is less useful because it has missed crucial deadlines. This will always be a dilemma in formative evaluation and it is perhaps best to recognise the tensions inherent in any reporting schedule so that expectations remain realistic. Making the tensions explicit for stakeholders will help them to attach appropriate weight to interim reports and to remain alert to the possibility of subsequent updating reports.

Including a dissemination schedule in your initial evaluation plan can help to ensure that this activity is allocated sufficient time and attention. Providing evaluation feedback in stages, to meet the immediate needs of stakeholders, should be balanced with recognition of the time required for adequate data processing and interpretation, and writing well crafted reports. Disadvantages associated with staged feedback include: potential loss of an overview, a risk of overemphasising details in relation to larger-scale messages, and a risk of confu-sion or disappointment as early messages change in the light of subsequent data collection, analysis and interpretation.

On the other hand, in participative evaluation designs, such as action research (outlined in Chapter nine), rapid cycles of provisional feedback and discursive development are at the heart of the curriculum development and evaluation process. This means less discomfort with evolving evaluation narratives and a correspondingly evolving interprofessional education initiative.

It is good practice for staged feedback to be clearly marked with its date of issue so that anyone in receipt of multiple reports can identify the appropriate historical sequence. The degree to which any particular report represents early findings, interim analyses, or a more nuanced account of particular facets of the interprofessional education should be made clear in the introduction. This will orientate the recipients to the status of the material presented and help them to assess the validity of drawing particular inferences. Readers (or listeners) can then make informed decisions that draw upon evidence from the evaluation reports.

Sharing interim evaluation findings with stakeholders is also an important part of the process of forming a well-evidenced and critical interpretation of the evaluation data. Presenting and explaining analyses to others helps the evaluation team to think systematically and critically about the data and the evaluation interpretations. Crystallising thoughts in this way is valuable to the ongoing evaluation. Reactions to interim reports help analysis and interpretation further by incorporating a wider range of perspectives and correcting mistakes and often elicit new data. Sharing interim findings assists the evaluation team to think critically about the progress of the evaluation, make changes where necessary and helps to ensure that recommendations are well-focused and realistic.

Sharing your evaluation findings more widely

Once the needs of the immediate stakeholders have been met it is time to give your attention to sharing your evaluation findings more widely. Although external reporting is another task for the curriculum development group and the evaluation team (and therefore an additional cost) external reporting is very important.[1] You will want to celebrate successes and other people will be interested to hear about them. Although you may feel less enthusiastic about sharing things that did not go well, these may be the very areas where there is most to be gained from your experience. It is not a good use of resources for everyone developing interprofessional education to learn only from their own mistakes.

The critical thinking required for preparing your evaluation account for external dissemination and feedback from peers adds further to the sharpening of analyses, interpretations and recommendations that we discussed in the previous section in relation to internal stakeholder feedback. Through external dissemination you may benefit from the insights of peer reviewers appointed by journal editors, or by the organisation that will publish your evaluation report. Presenting your evaluation at conferences or other meetings will often allow you to benefit from a discussion with interested peers. Even web-mounted reports can be linked to prompts that elicit feedback or encourage electronic discussion.

External evaluation accounts have an additional specialist audience within the interprofessional education community: other teams of evaluators. They will be keen to see not only the details of the interprofessional education that was evaluated, the evaluation findings and recommendations, but also a critical account of the evaluation design and execution. Such accounts promote the exchange of ideas and testing of evaluation assumptions and arguments. Interprofessional education

---

[1] With all your reporting it is important to pay attention to research governance frameworks and research ethics requirements. The evaluation of interprofessional education is almost always human subjects research, see Chapter ten.

is a complex initiative within complex environments: and often a long-term investment. This makes it particularly difficult to evaluate. Colleagues working in the
same field are likely to be interested in studying your evaluation questions and
design, and learning about the evaluation's processes and pitfalls.

Linking your evaluation to wider contexts or debates

In Chapter nine, under the heading of securing sufficient preliminary understanding, we discussed reviewing others' evaluations of interprofessional education,
and reading about the evaluation methodologies and theoretical perspectives that
may be relevant for understanding interprofessional education. This was to
enable new work to benefit from earlier insights and developments. The data
analysis and interpretation stage of your evaluation will also benefit from re-
course to the wider literature, policy and practice. You will need to summarise
facts, opinions and recommendations for use by those in the immediate setting,
but your evaluation will be more insightful and possibly more useful to a wider
range of readers if its findings and interpretations are explicitly linked to debates
and ideas beyond the local evaluation context. For example, when discussing the
limited impact of implementing two new interprofessional initiatives in stroke
care (see Box 11.6.), Gibbon *et al.* (2002) discussed the problem of trying to meet
UK national policy requirements for delivering effective collaboration, without
any guidance on the types of interprofessional initiatives needed to achieve this
aim. Another example is provided by Richardson & Cooper (2003) in their
evaluation of the use of information technology, via the Internet, to develop a
virtual interprofessional community among research students. In providing a
more in-depth insight into their findings, the authors discussed the implications
of their work in relation to Lave & Wenger's (1991) 'communities of practice'
theory of learning.

Audience and purpose

When communicating the learning from evaluations of interprofessional education two aspects are key: the purpose of each presentation and its intended
audience. Key questions to ask yourself include:

- Who are you trying to inform and what messages are you trying to get across?
- What type of communication is your intended audience used to?
- What is the likely epistemological stance of your intended audience(s)?

These questions can be particularly challenging in the context of interprofessional
education. The range of stakeholders can be particularly wide and professions

have developed different ways of 'knowing' and constructing arguments (that is, different epistemological stances, and perhaps ontological differences too). As we discussed in Chapter two, evidence and effectiveness are both contested concepts. A one-size-fits-all approach to reporting your evaluation may mean that several key audiences pay it scant attention.

The British Educational Research Association (BERA, 2000, p. 2) offered a useful 'pyramid model' of connected writings as good practice in the dissemination of educational research (see Figure 13.1). The pyramid's strata address the needs of different audiences. At its base is a 'full report'. This provides details of the design, execution and limitations of the research, an extended presentation and discussion of findings, and perhaps a range of recommendations for various stakeholder groups. The full report allows local stakeholders, concerned with development and delivery, to identify the finer points of your findings and apply these to their evolving interprofessional education. The full report also contains sufficient detail for those beyond the local context to evaluate the credibility of the evaluation and the strengths and weaknesses of the evaluated interprofessional education.

The next level within the pyramid model is peer-reviewed papers and articles. Publishing constraints mean that these will be quite short reports (perhaps 2000–3000 words). Nevertheless they will set your work in the context of the wider body of knowledge and experience in relation to interprofessional education. The text of these needs to be concise, clear and accurate. Comments that arise during the peer review process will help to sharpen your arguments and their presentation; and will play a gate-keeping role in relation to quality.

There are multiple audiences for papers and articles: those who develop and deliver interprofessional education, people with experience of interprofessional learning, people who develop and deliver education for a specific profession, health and social care practitioners, commissioners of professional and interprofessional education, people aiming to develop practice and services, policy makers, other evaluators and researchers. Students will also be part of this audience, reading and using your work to enhance their thinking and support their arguments. These audiences tend to browse in different types of journal, magazine and other news sources. The appropriate position for your paper or article depends upon its intended audience as well as upon its length, purpose and academic rigour. A large evaluation, with several strands to report, may result in a series of papers in a range of publications, each slanted towards the needs of a particular audience and aimed at communicating a particular message. Purposes and messages might include curriculum development (both profession-specific and interprofessional), practice development (in care settings, education

News report(s)
Professional report(s)
Peer-reviewed papers(s) and article(s)
Full report of the evaluation giving sufficient detail for replication and audit

Figure 13.1 Pyramid model of evaluation publications (adapted from BERA, 2000, p. 2).

delivery and evaluation), staff development for tutors and practice-based mentors who deliver interprofessional education, cost–benefit analyses, consideration of processes and outcomes (for the interprofessional education and for the evaluation), methodological development, theory building and hypothesis testing.

The pyramid model depicted in Figure 13.1 suggests that messages for managers, policy makers and practitioners may warrant a series of concise 'professional reports'. These would contain straightforward summaries of the interprofessional education, the evaluation and its findings; then give detailed attention to the professional, managerial or policy implications of the reported work. Professional reports guide readers in respect of the potential value of the work reported, suggesting how it might be used in similar or contrasting contexts.

News items and press releases feature at the apex of the pyramid. These draw attention to the professional reports, papers and fuller evaluation reports, in addition to publicising the interprofessional education itself. Attention to news items helps to ensure that your work will make a difference beyond its immediate context.

Fracturing the findings of an evaluation of interprofessional education by reporting separately to each participating profession undermines the collaborative endeavour, but for the evaluation to have been successful its messages need to reach and influence each group. This might be aided by sections within the full report that address the particular concerns of each participating profession, of managers, of funding organisations, and so on. Papers, articles and professional reports will be more clearly targeted at a particular audience, but can still retain a view of the whole through short summary sections or by cross-referencing to other publications.

Dissemination can encourage further collaboration and should lead to development. For this reason workshops are a popular and effective way of disseminating evaluation findings to targeted groups. The workshop format ensures that misconceptions can be addressed, alternative interpretations aired, practical applications discussed and action plans formulated.

Communicating clearly

Language

Clear communication is an important part of the effective dissemination and use of your evaluation findings and plain language plays an important role in that communication. Try to write simply and succinctly. The active voice (Many people reported...) is easier to read and more succinct than the passive voice (It was reported by many people that...). Unnecessary abbreviations and acronyms should be avoided, as should jargon. Necessary technical terms, definitions and important abbreviations or acronyms can be explained in a glossary. Gender-stereotyped language should be avoided: see the British Sociological Association's

(2003) guidelines on this. Always check your writing carefully for phrases or descriptions that may cause offence to particular individuals or groups.

Access to a good dictionary and other texts is essential. Examples are suggested in the further reading list at the end of this chapter and although some of these are aimed at students, their guidance is useful for writing evaluation reports. If your evaluation has taken a particular methodological stance, for example it is an ethnographic account of an interprofessional education initiative, then it would be wise to follow advice specific to writing up findings from that methodology (continuing with the example of ethnography, Hammersely & Atkinson, 1995, offer good advice). More generally, Dey (1993) has a chapter on producing an account of the analysis of qualitative data and Grbich (1999) looked at the presentation of data specifically for qualitative research in health. Robson (2002) discussed the reporting of different types of enquiry and Chapman (1996) showed how to present numerical findings effectively.

Of course, however clear your language not everyone will draw the same information and conclusions from your writing or verbal presentations. Reading and listening are active processes, and will be contextualised by the individual recipients of your work. Those who read or listen to what you have to say will judge its credibility and applicability from their own perspectives; they will bring differing stores of prior experience and knowledge to its interpretation.

Length and structure

In general, shorter is better and a clear structure aids communication. The following might help: informative headings and subheadings; and 'signposts' in the prose or presentation to tell people what to expect in subsequent sections, or to refer them back to a relevant passage that appeared earlier. Long reports benefit from summaries in each chapter, in addition to an executive summary and an abstract. Information that must be included for completeness but would interrupt the flow of your presentation can be placed in appendices to the written report, or in a handout to accompany a verbal presentation.

One useful way to think about structure is *description-analysis-interpretation*. Description tells people what existed and what was done. Analysis organises what was found and shows the relationships and pattern that emerged. Interpretation involves saying what you think the findings mean, how they relate to the work of others and how they should be used. It is easy for the evaluators to become enthralled by the description and analysis, but people interested in using the evaluation will probably focus more on the interpretation sections. Thus, it is important for evaluators to give sufficient attention to interpretation and suggestions for applying the findings.

Sometimes it is tempting to present a large quantity of description, some analysis and just a little interpretation. This can be driven by a desire to let the data speak for themselves or to encourage active processing by readers and alternative interpretations. Actually, data do not really speak for themselves.

They may appear to do so for the evaluators who have spent many weeks developing an understanding of the data set, seeing patterns and mulling over alternative interpretations. For the first-time reader vast tracts of description and quotation simply create overload. Evaluation users need evaluators to organise, distil, evaluate and interpret. That is part of an evaluator's role.

Most evaluations have to choose between a number of plausible structures for organising the findings and interpretations, including:

- Highlighting the perspectives and concerns of different stakeholders
- Dividing material according to the main categories that emerged in the findings
- Showing chronological development cycles
- Comparing and contrasting different sites or different types of data

The organisation of the text may serve to highlight a central event or process and show how different antecedents contributed and different outcomes emerged. Alternatively, it may set out a series of case studies that exhibit features you wish to draw out in the analysis and interpretation, or even start with outcomes and trace their antecedents and inter-relationships. There are many logical ways to tell a story. The choice depends on the audience and on the central messages of your evaluation.

Selecting content

The content of your report or presentation should be tailored to its audience and permitted length. The sections you select are likely to be a subset from the following list, which you will arrange in a sequence that is logical for the argument you are developing. Only a full evaluation report would have all of the sections in the list (see Figure 13.1).

- Title, preferably one that is both memorable and informative
- Authorship, departmental and institutional affiliation and a statement about any conflicts of interest
- Copyright information
- Tables of content, chapters, subsections, figures and tables
- Abstract and keywords, see below
- Acknowledgements, particularly for funding and listing any contributors who do not qualify for authorship
- Glossary
- An executive summary targeted on the needs of the intended audience(s)

Pages in the above sections are usually numbered with Roman numerals (i, ii, iii etc.), the ones below with Arabic numerals (1, 2, 3, etc.).

- Introduction, including an outline of the local context, summaries of the initial situation or problem and the purpose of the evaluation, with a list of the evaluation questions. This is also the place to give an outline of what is to follow.
- Background information, expanding on material in the introduction to describe relevant aspects of the local context and details of the interprofessional education; discussion of wider contexts including policy, practice development, previously published evaluations, the theoretical underpinnings of both the interprofessional education and evaluation methodology. This will need to be divided into several short sections.
- Literature review, if this has not been covered within the background information section. This will foreshadow your evaluation and set the interprofessional education initiative and its evaluation in a wider context. It should be succinct, but identify the most important prior work in the field, perhaps also drawing attention to contradictions and gaps. Subheadings can be used very effectively to highlight key themes within the literature. The aim is to synthesise and evaluate prior work: not simply to list and describe.
- An account of how the evaluation was conducted, paying attention to ethics, sampling, trustworthiness, methodological choices and methods of data collection and analysis, pragmatic decisions and a reflexive account of limitations.
- Findings, arranged under informative subheadings and illustrated with diagrams, tables, graphs and quotations as appropriate.
- Discussion and interpretation: this will elaborate on the findings and link your work to that of others.
- Conclusions, no more than are warranted by the preceding sections.
- Recommendations, not exceeding what is warranted by the preceding sections.
- References and/or a bibliography, and suggested further reading. These should be formatted in one of the standard ways, for example using the Harvard, Vancouver, American Psychological Association (APA) or Modern Language Association (MLA) referencing system. Journals, web publishers and organisations vary in their citation and reference requirements. Try to decide which one to use early in the writing process.
- Appendices, commonly including research instruments, data samples, details from the analysis, etc.

Specific audiences will expect particular styles. A sense of what is expected and what works well can be obtained by reading evaluation reports, papers and articles targeted at audiences similar to those you wish to address.

Journals provide detailed guidance on scope, length, format, structure and their peer-review process to authors who wish to submit papers or short reports. These instructions can usually be found both within the print version of any edition of the journal and (often in more detail) on the journal's website. Guidance on scope is particularly important since the editor will have to reject your paper, no matter how good, if it falls outside the scope of the journal. Matters of tone, style and 'hot topics' are best gleaned by reading several recent issues of the journal you are targeting. From time to time journals publish useful articles to help authors submit well structured papers of the required standard for publication. Examples include: Newell (2001), Belgrave *et al.* (2002), Burnard (2004) and Newton *et al.* (2004); and the *Journal of Postgraduate Medicine* has lots of information for writers on their website (see further reading).

Inclusion and exclusion

Evaluations quickly gather an overwhelming amount of data. You will not be able to present everything; and not everything will be important and useful. Concepts, patterns and relationships that are important to understanding the findings need to be presented and explained. Interprofessional education evaluators will not have the luxury of the time required for purist grounded analyses that account for every scrap of data. Some minor points or deviations will almost certainly need to be excluded to create a coherent report that delivers key messages for development, whilst avoiding excessive length.

The amount of evidence and detail from the evaluation data set presented should be sufficient to make your report readable and believable. Quotations that clarify and substantiate categories or points are useful and bring a report alive. Be guided by the thought that nobody else is likely to be quite as fascinated by your raw data as you are. A small number of well-chosen quotes always go down better than lengthy passages that can detract from your central message and will help people to understand and apply the evaluation findings.

Tables, graphs and diagrams can summarise information or ideas very succinctly and may be better remembered than the prose. When well-chosen and well-presented they are an asset, highlighting key features of your findings or message. These need to be as uncluttered as possible, and adequately labelled to permit accurate interpretation. Be wary of using any that place undue emphasis on minor points or distract readers from the main messages. Chapman (1996) offered a wealth of sound advice for the presentation of quantitative data and Bogdan & Bicklen (1992) have a useful chapter on writing up qualitative research for education.

Mode of presentation

Written reports of various types are the most common format for sharing evaluation findings. Verbal presentations are also very common, although usually augmented by some form of written summary. Appearances before various committees, conference presentations, workshops and media appearances may all feature. More innovative formats include drama, poetry, pictorial art, sculpture and video presentations. These can be very powerful means of communicating your message, although they can be limited in relation to balance, emphasis and coverage. They usually augment, rather than replace, traditional written or spoken reports. Learning materials for students or staff development materials may be another useful way to package the learning from your evaluation.

Abstracts and keywords

Abstracts are a particularly important aspect of written reports because they may be the only part of your evaluation that is freely and easily accessible to people searching for useful information and ideas by conducting a search of a bibliographic database or the World Wide Web. Abstract submissions are also the most common mode of selecting contributions to conferences and other professional meetings. People will often judge the relevance and importance of your work from its abstract alone. This means that it is important to convey as accurately as brevity permits, the boundaries and context of your work, the approach to enquiry that was used, and an indication of the results, findings, claims or recommendations arising from your work. Adding keywords to your abstract, especially keywords extracted from the thesaurus of one of the main bibliographic databases, will ensure that search engines locate and display your article when people search for similar or related material.

Boundaries and limitations

Evaluation reports should make clear what they are reporting and what they are not reporting; also what the evaluation addressed and what it did not address. In full reports this is likely to comprise a clear statement of the evaluation questions and aims, and its boundaries. There is also likely to be a limitations section that discusses what was noticed but could not be followed up, any aims that were not fully realised, known or probable bias, and the limitations inherent in the particular approach to enquiry adopted (for example aspects of validation and generalisability). If certain parts of the evaluation did not perform well or go according to plan it is appropriate to reflect on this and draw out lessons for future work. In shorter reports this discussion will necessarily be curtailed, but readers should still be clear about what is being reported, what is being claimed, and on what grounds.

Recommendations and options

Recommendations are an extension of the interpretation phase of evaluation. They need to be grounded by an appreciation of what is practical and acceptable; a task made easier by ongoing communication between the evaluation team and the stakeholders throughout the life of the evaluation. Recommendations need to be highlighted to the appropriate audiences (for example policy makers, service commissioners, education commissioners, professional bodies, mentors in practice, university tutors, etc.). Recommendations that are too expensive or politically unpalatable are unlikely to be implemented. Nevertheless, they might serve as markers for the longer term. In this case, it might be helpful to separate recommendations that are thought applicable to different time horizons (for example short, medium and long term).

Sometimes options may be sketched out representing alternative future scenarios. These will be most useful if there is some discussion of each option's likely implications in terms of implementation needs and predicted outcomes. In this way you show how you think your evaluation findings might be used.

Barriers to using your evaluation findings

There will be many barriers to the implementation of your evaluation findings. Some may be beyond your control but many can be influenced, to some extent. It is helpful to consider the evaluation team in partnership with the commissioners of the evaluation and the developers of the interprofessional education. All these partners want the evaluation effort to be worthwhile and to produce evidence-based improvement or more informed continuation.

The most controllable barrier is where people fail to understand your findings or are unsure of how these might be applied. Ongoing communication with stakeholders throughout the evaluation and clear well-targeted reporting (the foci of most of this chapter) are the main means of avoiding such problems. For example, you could demonstrate that your recommendations are practical by providing some realistic suggestions of how they might be implemented. Interprofessional education is a complex initiative and it is likely that the evaluation team will be communicating complexity and subtlety in preference to strong, simple messages. However, the people trying to implement the evaluation findings need reasonably strong and reasonably straightforward messages if they are to act. The evaluation team needs to set out the stronger messages from the evaluation and to clearly indicate the perceived limits of their applicability.

Evaluation findings will not be used if they do not reach and convince decision makers and opinion leaders. This means communicating with them in formats that they will access and in harmony with their decision-making timetables. Targeted feedback to particular decision makers at particular times, based on the firm foundation of the full evaluation report, is an important part of increasing the chance of your findings being used. Evaluators need to understand the literature relating to dissemination of innovation and theories of change. The UK Higher Education Academy (2004) offers some overviews of different dimensions of change aimed at supporting the promotion and embedding of good practice and facilitating change in higher education (see further reading at the end of this chapter). It is also helpful to have an understanding of the history of change and decision-making processes in the local context.

Your evaluation findings may upset a key stakeholder who then tries to block its dissemination and implementation. As we noted in Chapter ten, evaluators cannot expect to be popular with everybody or popular all of the time. Ongoing communication with individuals who feel threatened is very important. Be alert to the potential to allay their fears and reach a compromise. It may be that the evaluation team made a mistake in their analysis and interpretation which can be corrected at an early stage. It may be that the evaluation challenges deeply held beliefs and time-honoured practices. Inviting discussion of staged feedback to stakeholders helps people to identify and discuss sensitive areas. Working with people to support them in experimenting with new ways of working may also be important.

As we discussed in Chapter ten, key champions and gate-keepers may move posts, leaving the evaluation team with no one to report to, or having to forge new relationships. New significant post holders may have other priorities and will certainly need time to catch up with the development and evaluation of the interprofessional education that you know so well. They will need individual briefings as soon as the priorities of their roles permit.

A changing political climate at local levels, or more generally, may mean that the priorities of the original interprofessional education development and its evaluation no longer match the priorities of the day. In this situation, sound work is often ignored because other priorities are more pressing or attractive. It may be possible for you to show that your work does have some bearing on the new priorities. In some cases this may only require a different form of presentation; in others a return to analysis may be signalled. In the unlikely event that your evaluation cannot be linked to today's concerns it is still worth producing a careful and succinct report in a format that will be available for many years to come (perhaps a peer-reviewed journal article and an archived full report). Political priorities often feel cyclical. It could just be a matter of time until your work is important, provided it is of a sufficiently high standard to withstand the test of time.

Lack of resources (money, time, space or even enthusiasm) will slow or halt the implementation of your evaluation findings. Emphasising practical recommendations will help to guard against this, as will helping stakeholders to prioritise recommendations and separating recommendations into the different time frames, as we suggested above.

Lack of reward for the effort of using your findings will discourage their use: it is rational not to do work that will bring no reward or even negative consequences. Sometimes this is an organisational matter, beyond the control of the evaluation team, but occasionally the evaluation team can influence by explaining more thoroughly the benefits that people can expect from using the evaluation findings.

Conclusion

Evaluations should be useful to local stakeholders and the wider interprofessional education community. To achieve this, findings need to be communicated in a clear and timely fashion, and linked to wider debates. The form of reporting should match different stakeholder groups' needs and expectations. While descriptions of what was done and what was found are important, the main contribution of an evaluation is to interpret findings. Evaluators can help the stakeholders to take appropriate action by making practical recommendations.

Not everything that can be evaluated is important and not everything that is important can be captured within a particular evaluation design. Tacit and craft knowledge, and complex social interactions can be overlooked in evaluations because they are difficult to capture. However, we should strive to illuminate their presence because they exert a powerful influence on the effectiveness of interprofessional education.

Key points

- Evaluations should be useful to stakeholders. Usefulness has several facets, including the focus of reports, their style, length and timing.
- Begin dissemination early and continue throughout the life of the evaluation.
- Ensure adequate resources for dissemination by scheduling interim and summary reports to a variety of stakeholders in the evaluation plan.
- Well conducted dissemination will leave participants well disposed towards future evaluations and engender goodwill and trust in other evaluation settings.
- Evaluation findings need to be shared beyond the immediate context, and one-size-fits-all dissemination is ineffective. Expect to write several documents targeted to the needs, concerns and standpoints of different stakeholder groups.
- Seek to connect your local evaluation findings to wider contexts and debates.

Further reading

Barrass, R. (1995) *Students Must Write: A Guide to Better Writing in Coursework and Examinations*. 2nd edn. Routledge, London.

British Educational Research Association (2000) *Good Practice in Educational Research Writing*. BERA, Southwell.

British Sociological Association (2003) Professional standards: authorship guidelines, anti-sexist, anti-racist, ablist and non-disablist language. Available from:
  http://www.britsoc.co.uk/bsaweb.php?area = item1&link_id = 15
  (accessed 7 July 2004).

Burnard, P. (2004) Writing a qualitative research report. *Nurse Education Today*, **24**, 174–9.

Chalker, S. & Weiner, E.S.C. (1998) *Oxford Dictionary of English Grammar*. Oxford Paperbacks, Oxford.

Higher Education Academy (2004) *Facilitating Change*. Available from: http://www. heacademy.ac.uk/1745.htm (accessed 19 November 2004).

International Committee of Medical Journal Editors (2003) Uniform requirements for manuscripts. Available from: http://www.icmje.org/index.html (accessed July 7 2004).

Journal of Postgraduate Medicine. Resources for contributors. Available from: http://www.jpgmonline.com/contributor2.asp (accessed 7 July 2004).

National Education Research Forum (2000) *The Impact of Educational Research on Policy and Practice: Sub-group Report*. National Education Research Forum, London. Available from: www.nerf-uk.org/software/impact_report.doc?version = 1 (accessed 5 June 2004).

Weiner, E.S.C. & Delahunty, A. (eds) (1994) *Oxford Guide to English Usage: The Essential Guide to Correct English*. Oxford University Press, Oxford.

Young, P. (1996) *The Art and Science of Writing: A Handbook for Health Science Students*. Chapman & Hall, London.

Endnote: Drawing the Threads Together

Finally, we draw together the three distinctive parts of the book in a set of key messages that relate to our two themes or master narratives.

(1) The *practice* of developing, delivering and evaluating diverse curricula underpinned by the principles of interprofessional education.
(2) *Effectiveness* and what this means in the development, delivery and evaluation of interprofessional education.

There are three checklists covering the various activities required to develop, deliver and evaluate an effective interprofessional initiative. First, though, a reminder about the four objectives we set out in Chapter one and the overall structure of the book.

Objectives

(1) To guide trainers and educators through process of developing, delivering and evaluating interprofessional education for health and social care: whether as an entirely new development or by modification of existing provision.
(2) To draw attention to the current practice of interprofessional education, nationally and internationally, through examples and research-based models.
(3) To discuss the key organisational and resource (financial and human) factors underpinning the successful delivery of effective interprofessional education.
(4) To describe evaluation approaches and processes appropriate for different models of interprofessional education and provide guidance for the use of these in everyday practice.

Structure

To meet these objectives we mapped and discussed, in three separate (but over-lapping) parts, a range of core concepts and issues related to the development, delivery and evaluation of an interprofessional initiative. In Section I (Chapters one and two) we examined a number of the fundamental concepts underpinning interprofessional education: its definition, aims, motives and uses within health and social care and explored the notion of effectiveness and its application in interprofessional education.

In Section II (Chapters three to eight) we focused on the issues and processes associated with planning and implementing an interprofessional initiative within your local context. We described a range of key features related to these activities. These included: the presage-process-product model to help to focus your think-ing; group work issues for the individuals involved in planning an initiative; ideas for developing suitable interprofessional curricula and the assessment of learning on an interprofessional initiative.

In Section III (Chapters nine to thirteen) we turned to the designs, methodolo-gies and methods that you can draw upon in planning a sound evaluation of interprofessional education. We discussed key issues related to undertaking any educational evaluation, such as ethics and governance, accessing the evaluation site and the resources required to successfully complete this work. This Section also showed the range of dissemination routes available to you to enable key messages from your evaluation to be communicated to an audience of peers, managers, policy makers and service users.

Checklist for Section I: fundamental ideas and issues

- Interprofessional education (like all education) should strive to achieve posi-tive change and maximise positive, whilst minimising negative, learning.
- Interprofessional education aims to promote interprofessional collaboration and enhance professional practice. Its aims are to improve the effectiveness of care, stakeholders' perceptions of care and practitioners' working lives.
- Interprofessional education needs to be effective for its participants. As such, it delivers positive outcomes, at an acceptable cost, without unacceptable side effects.
- Developing an effective interprofessional education initiative is difficult. The notion of effectiveness is complex and contestable. Clarity of the definition and use of the concept of effectiveness is essential when planning an interprofes-sional education initiative.
- Interprofessional education should not be viewed as a one-off experience of learning how to collaborate; rather it is a continuous part of a health or social care practitioner's professional development.

Checklist for Section II: development and delivery issues and processes

- Interaction between participants is central to interprofessional education. This marks it out from multi-professional education, where there is no planned interactive learning.
- The use of the presage-process-product model can help to structure discussions about the different elements in the development of an interprofessional education initiative.
- Time should be taken to explore and understand the nature of the collaborative relationships between those who develop and deliver an interprofessional initiative. This will ensure that you and your colleagues can work together in an effective and mutually satisfying manner.
- Enthusiasm and commitment from individuals involved in the planning and delivering of an interprofessional initiative (including senior level champions) are essential ingredients in any initiative's success.
- Members of the planning team require a clear plan of the joint work they undertake. The selection of a suitable curriculum (one that meets the needs of the local context) and the delivery of a pilot initiative are important elements in the successful development and delivery of interprofessional education.
- Learner motivation and resistance are two key and interlinking issues for learners. Time spent on ways to maximise learner motivation, whilst minimising any resistance to interprofessional learning and developing an effective assessment strategy, should help.
- Interprofessional facilitation is a demanding task. Teaching staff will need training opportunities to meet the demands of their work on your interprofessional initiative.
- Successful accreditation of your interprofessional initiative (if required) requires good preparation. It should be as inclusive as possible, embracing a range of perspectives, such as the learners, teachers, administrators and managers.

Checklist for Section III: evaluation planning, fieldwork and dissemination

- A sound evaluation depends upon developing answerable evaluation questions that are informed by negotiation with stakeholders and take into account the evaluation context.
- Once a set of answerable questions has been identified, the next task is to select appropriate research design, methodology and data collection methods. This work is fundamental to the planning of an achievable evaluation.
- When your evaluation plan is ready, the next step is to calculate the resources required to implement it and identify whether these are available. If

your resources are less than your plan requires, then replanning is the way forward.

- Time needs to be taken to ensure that your evaluation plan complies with all relevant research governance requirements (for example ethical committee approval, registration of project). The aim is for good practice in the conduct and dissemination of your evaluation.
- Evaluation is a dynamic process, your enquiry will benefit from a regular review of its progress and, when circumstances demand, a rethink and replan.
- Dissemination is essential throughout the life of the evaluation. The selection of how to approach this (using, for example, presentations, internal reports, peer-reviewed journal papers) depends on the information and communication needs of your different stakeholders.

Final thoughts

These checklists provide you with a distillation of the elements involved in developing, delivering and evaluating your interprofessional initiative. They are not meant as a substitute for engagement with the relevant chapters with a view to linking the concepts, issues and approaches we have written about to the constraints and opportunities of your local context. This will optimise the enjoyment and effectiveness of your work of developing, delivering and evaluating interprofessional education.

We wish you every success.

References

Alderson, P., Farsides, B. & Williams, C. (2002) Examining ethics in practice: health service professionals' evaluations of in-hospital ethics seminars. *Nursing Ethics*, **9** (5), 508–521.

Anderson, N. & West, M. (1994) *The Team Climate Inventory: Manual and Users' Guide*. ASE Press, Windsor.

Anderson, N. & West, M. (1998) Measuring climate for work group innovation: development and validation of the team climate inventory. *Journal of Organisational Behavior*, **19**, 235–58.

Areskog, N.-H. (1995) The Linköping case: a transition from traditional to innovative medical school. *Medical Teacher*, **17** (4), 371–6.

Argyris, C. (1990) *Overcoming Organisational Defenses: Facilitating Organisational Learning*. Allyn & Bacon, Boston, Mass.

Atwal, A. (2002) A world apart: how occupational therapists, nurses and care managers perceive each other in acute health care. *British Journal of Occupational Therapy*, **65** (7), 446–52.

Baker, B. & Hunt, H. (2002) Discuss critical path analysis. Available from: http://www.mis.coventry.ac.uk/~nhunt/cpa (accessed 5 July 2004).

Bales, R. (1976) *Interaction Process Analysis: a Method for the Study of Small Groups*. University of Chicago, Chicago.

Bales, R. & Cohen, S. (1979) *SYMLOG: a System For Multiple Level Observation of Groups*. Free Press, New York.

Barnes, D., Carpenter, J. & Dickinson, C. (2000) Interprofessional education for community mental health: attitudes to community care and professional stereotypes. *Social Work Education*, **19** (6), 565–83.

Barr, H. (1996) Ends and means in interprofessional education: towards a typology. *Education for Health*, **9** (3), 341–52.

Barr, H. (2002) *Interprofessional Education: Today, Yesterday and Tomorrow*. Occasional Paper No. 1. The Learning and Teaching Support Network for Health Sciences and Practice, London.

Barr, H. (2003) *Ensuring Quality in Interprofessional Education*. Centre for Advancement of Interprofessional Education Bulletin 22, London.

Barr, H., Freeth, D., Hammick, M., Koppel, I. & Reeves, S. (2000) *Evaluations of Interprofessional Education: A UK Review for Health and Social Care*. CAIPE/BERA, London. Available from: http://www.caipe.org.uk/publications.html (accessed 14 June 2003).

Barr, H., Koppel, I., Reeves, S., Hammick, M. & Freeth, D. (2005) *Effective Interprofessional Education: Argument, Assumption and Evidence*. Blackwell Publishing, Oxford.

Barrett, G., Greenwood, R. & Ross, K. (2003) Integrating interprofessional education into ten health and social care programmes. *Journal of Interprofessional Care*, **17** (3), 203–310.

Becker, H. (1970) *Sociological Work: Method and Substance*. Transaction Books, New Jersey.

Becker, H. (1986) *Writing for Social Scientists: How to Start and Finish your Thesis, Book or Article*. University of Chicago Press, Chicago.

Belbin, M. (1993) *Team Roles at Work*. Butterworth-Heinmann, Oxford.

Belbin, R. (1981) *Management Teams: Why they Succeed or Fail*. Butterworth-Heinmann, Oxford.

Belgrave, L., Zablotsky, D. & Guadango, M. (2002) How do we talk to each other? Writing qualitative research for quantitative readers. *Qualitative Health Research*, **12** (10), 1427–39.

Berman, S., Miller, C., Rosen, C. & Bicchieri, S. (2000) Assessment training and team functioning for children with disabilities. *Archives of Physical Medicine and Rehabilitation*, **81** (5), 628–33.

Bezzina, P., Keogh, J. & Keogh, M. (1998) Teaching primary health care: an interdisciplinary approach. *Nurse Education Today*, **18** (1), 36–45.

Biggs, J. (1993) From theory to practice: a cognitive systems approach. *Higher Education Research and Development*, **12**, 73–85.

Biggs, J. (2003) *Teaching for Quality Learning at University*. 2nd edn. SRHE & Open University Press, Buckingham.

Billet, S. (1996) Towards a model of workplace learning: the learning curriculum. *Studies in Higher Education*, **18** (1), 43–58.

Blaikie, N. (2000) *Designing Social Research: the Logic of Anticipation*. Polity Press, Cambridge.

Blaxer, L., Hughes, C. & Tight, M. (1996) *How to Research*. Open University Press, Milton Keynes.

Bluespruce, J., Dodge, W., Grothaus, L., *et al.* (2001) HIV prevention in primary care: impact of a clinical initiative. *AIDS Patient Care & Studies*, **15** (5), 243–53.

Bogdan, R. C. & Bicklen, S. J. (1992) *Qualitative Research for Education: an Introduction to Theory and Methods*. 2nd edn. Allyn and Bacon, Boston.

Boud, D. & Feletti, G. (1998) *The Challenge of Problem-based Learning*. 2nd edn. Kogan Page, London.

Brennan, J. & Shah, T. (2000) *Managing Quality in Higher Education, an International Perspective on Institutional Assessment and Change*. OECD, SRHE, Open University Press, Buckingham.

British Educational Research Association (2000) *Good Practice in Educational Research Writing*. British Educational Research Association, Southwell.

British Sociological Association (2003) Professional standards: authorship guidelines, anti-sexist, anti-racist ablist and non-disablist language. Available from: http://www.britsoc.co.uk/bsaweb.php?area=item1& link_id=15 (accessed 7 July 2004).

Brockbank, A. & McGill, I. (1998) *Facilitating Reflective Learning in Higher Education*. SRHE and Open University Press, Buckingham.

Brown, G., Bull, J. & Pendlebury, M. (1997) *Assessing Student Learning in Higher Education*. Routledge, London.

Brown, V. & Adkins, B. (1989) A comprehensive training program for multidisciplinary treatment plans. *Journal of Nursing Staff Development*, **5** (1), 25–9.

Bruner, J. (1977) *The Process of Education*. Revised edn. Harvard University Press, Mass.

Burnard, P. (2004) Writing a qualitative research report. *Nurse Education Today*, **24**, 174–9.

CAIPE (1997) *Interprofessional Education – a Definition*. CAIPE Bulletin. Centre for Advancement of Interprofessional Education, London.

Carpenter, J. (1995a) Interprofessional education for medical and nursing students: evaluation of a programme. *Medical Education*, **29** (4), 265–72.

Carpenter, J. (1995b) Doctors and nurses: stereotype and stereotype change in interprofessional education. *Journal of Interprofessional Care*, **9**, 151–62.

Carpenter, J. & Hewstone, M. (1996) Shared learning for doctors and social workers: evaluation of a programme. *British Journal of Social Work*, **26** (2), 239–57.

Carr, E., Brockbank, K. & Barrett, R. (2003) Improving pain management through interprofessional education: evaluation of a pilot project. *Learning in Health and Social Care*, **2**, 6–17.

Cashman, S., Reudy, P., Cody, K. & Lemay, C. (2004) Developing and measuring progress toward collaborative, integrated, interdisciplinary health care teams. *Journal of Interprofessional Care*, **18**, 183–96.

Chapman, M. (1996) *Plain Figures*. The Stationery Office Books, London.

Chopra, A. (1999) *Managing the People Side of Innovation: Eight Rules for Engaging Minds and Hearts*. Kumerian Press, West Hertford, Conn.

Clarke, A. & Dawson, R. (1999) *Evaluation Research: an Introduction to Principles, Methods and Practice*. Sage, London.

Clay, M., Lilley, S., Boree, K. & Harris, J. (1999) Applying adult education principles to the design of preceptor development program. *Journal of Interprofessional Care*, **13**, 405–415.

Cleghorn, G. & Baker, G. (2000) What faculty need to learn about improvement and how to teach it to others. *Journal of Interprofessional Care*, **14** (2), 147–59.

Clemmer, T., Spuhler, V., Oniki, T. & Horn, S. (1999) Results of a collaborative quality improvement program on outcomes and costs in a tertiary critical care unit. *Critical Care Medicine*, **27** (9), 1768–74.

Cohen, L., Manion, L. & Morrison, K. (2000) *Research Methods in Education*. 5th edn. Routledge Falmer, London.

Cook, S. & Drusin, R. (1995) Revisiting interdisciplinary education: one way to build an ark. *Nursing & Health Care Perspectives on Community*, **16**, 260–64.

Cornish, P., Church, E., Callanan, T., Bethune, C., Robbins, C. & Miller, R. (2003) Rural interdisciplinary mental health teambuilding via satellite: a demonstration project. *Telemedicine Journal & E-Health*, **9** (1), 63–71.

COT/CSLT/CSP (College of Occupational Therapists/College of Speech and Language Therapists/Chartered Society of Physiotherapists) (1993) *Promoting Collaborative Practice*. College of Occupational Therapists/College of Speech and Language Therapists/Chartered Society of Physiotherapists, London.

Cox, S., Wilcock, P. & Young, J. (1999) Improving the repeat prescribing process in a busy general practice: a study using continuous quality improvement methodology. *Quality in Health Care*, **8**, 119–25.

Crow, J. & Smith, L. (2003) Co-teaching in health and social care. *Journal of Interprofessional Care*, **17**, 43–55.

Davis, M. & Harden, R. (2003) Planning and implementing an undergraduate medical curriculum: the lessons learned. *Medical Teacher*, **25**, 596–608.

Degeling, P., Maxwell, S., Iedema, R. & Hunter, D.J. (2004) Making clinical governance work. *British Medical Journal*, **329**, 679–81.

Denscombe, M. (1998) *The Good Research Guide: for Small-scale Research Projects*. Open University Press, Buckingham.

Denzin, N. & Lincoln, Y. (eds) (1998) *The Landscape of Qualitative Research: Theories and Issues*. Sage, London.

Denzin, N. & Lincoln, Y. (eds) (2000) *Handbook of Qualitative Research*. 2nd edn. Sage, London.

Denzin, N. & Lincoln, Y. (eds) (2003) *Strategies of Qualitative Inquiry*. 2nd edn. Sage, London.

Department of Health and Social Security (1974) *The Joseph Report*. HMSO, London.

Department of Health (1998) *A First Class Service: Quality in the New NHS*. Department of Health, London.

Department of Health (2001) *Working Together, Learning Together: a Framework for Lifelong Learning for the NHS*. Department of Health, London.

Department of Health (2002) *NHS Dentistry: Options for Change*. Department of Health, London.

Dey, I. (1993) *Qualitative Data Analysis: A User Friendly Guide for Social Scientists*. Routledge, London.

Dienst, E. & Byl, N. (1981) Evaluation of an educational program in health care teams. *Journal of Community Health*, **6** (4), 282–98.

Doyle, M., Earnshaw, P. & Galloway, A. (2003) Developing, delivering and evaluating interprofessional clinical risk training in mental health services. *Psychiatric Bulletin*, **27**, 73–6.

Eby, M. (2000) Understanding professional development. In: *Critical Practice in Health and Social Care*. A. Brechin, H. Brown, M. Eby (eds) pp. 48–69. Sage, London.

Edwards, H., Baume, D. & Webb, G. (eds) (2003) *Staff and Educational Development*. Kogan Page, London.

Engeström, Y. (1999) Expansive visibilisation of work: an activity-theoretical perspective. *Computer Supported Cooperative Work*, **8**, 63–93.

Fallsberg, M. & Hammar, M. (2000) Strategies and focus at an integrated, interprofessional training ward. *Journal of Interprofessional Care*, **14** (4), 337–50.

Farrell, M., Ryan, S. & Langrick, B. (2001a) Breaking bad news within a paediatric setting: an evaluation report of a collaborative workshop to support health professionals. *Journal of Advanced Nursing*, **36** (6), 765–75.

Farrell, M., Schmitt, M. & Heinemann, G. (2001b) Informal roles and the stages of interdisciplinary team development. *Journal of Interprofessional Care*, **15**, 281–95.

Fink, A. (ed.) (1995) *The Survey Kit*. Sage, London.

Freeth, D., Hammick, M., Koppel, I., Reeves, S. & Barr, H. (2002) *A Critical Review of Evaluations of Interprofessional Education*. The Learning and Teaching Support Network for Health Sciences and Practice, London.

Freeth, D. & Nicol, M. (1998) Learning clinical skills: an interprofessional approach. *Nurse Education Today*, **18** (6), 455–61.

Freeth, D. & Reeves, S. (2004) Learning to work together: using the presage, process, product (3P) model to highlight decisions and possibilities. *Journal of Interprofessional Care*, **18** (1), 43–56.

Funnell, P. (1995) Exploring the value of interprofessional shared learning. In: *Interprofessional Relations in Health Care* (eds K. Soothill, L. Mackay & C. Webb), pp. 163–71. Edward Arnold, London.

Gelmon, S., White, A., Carlson, L. & Norman, L. (2000) Making organisational change to achieve improvement and interprofessional learning: perspectives from health professions educators. *Journal of Interprofessional Care*, **12** (3), 131–46.

Gibbon, B., Watkins, C., Barer, D., *et al.* (2002) Can staff attitudes to teamworking in stroke care be improved? *Journal of Advanced Nursing*, **40** (1), 105–111.

Gill, J. & Ling, J. (1995) Interprofessional shared learning: a curriculum for collaboration. In: *Interprofessional Relations in Health Care* (eds. K. Soothill, L. Mackay, & C. Webb) pp. 172–93. Edward Arnold, London.

Gomm, R., Hammersley, M. & Foster, P. (eds) (2000) *Case Study Method: Key Issues, Key Texts*. Sage, London.

Gorard, S. (2001) *Quantitative Methods in Educational Research: the Role of Numbers Made Easy*. Continuum, London.

Gottlieb, L. D., Roer, D., Jega, K., *et al.* (1996) Clinical pathways for pneumonia: development, implementation and initial experience. *Best Practices and Benchmarking in Healthcare*, **1** (5), 262–5.

Grbich, C. (1999) *Qualitative Research in Health: An Introduction*. Sage, Thousand Oaks, California.

Guest, C., Smith, L., Bradshaw, M. & Hardcastle, W. (2002) Facilitating interprofessional learning for medical and nursing students in clinical practice. *Learning in Health and Social Care*, **1**, 132–8.

Hammersley, M. & Atkinson, P. (1995) *Ethnography: Principles in Practice*. 2nd edn. Routledge, London.

Hammond, S. (1998) *The Thin Book of Appreciative Inquiry*. 2nd edn. Thin Book Publishing Co. Bend, Oreg.

Hart, E. & Bond, M. (1995) *Action Research for Health and Social Care: a Guide to Practice*. Open University Press, Milton Keynes.

Hayward, K., Powell, L. & McRoberts, J. (1996) Changes in student perceptions of interdisciplinary practice in the rural setting. *Journal of Allied Health*, **25** (4), 315–27.

Health Canada (2003) First Ministers' Accord on Health Care Renewal. Available from: www.hc-sc.gc.ca/english/hca2003/accord.html (accessed 14 June 2004).

Heinemann, G. & Zeiss, A. (2002) *Team Performance in Health Care: Assessment and Measurment*. Kluwer, New York.

Henry, G. (1990) *Practical Sampling*. Sage, London.

Higher Education Academy (2004) *Facilitating Change*. Available from: http://www.heacademy.ac.uk/1745 (accessed 19 November 2004).

Hind, M., Norman, I, Cooper, S., *et al.* (2003) Interprofessional perceptions of health care students. *Journal of Interprofessional Care*, **17**, 21–34.

Hook, A. & Lawson-Porter, A. (2003) The development and evaluation of a fieldwork educator's training programme for allied health professionals. *Medical Teacher*, **25**, 527–36.

Horbar, J. D., Rogowski, J., Plsek, P. E., *et al.* (2001) Collaborative quality improvement for neonatal intensive care. NIC/Q Project Investigators of the Vermont Oxford Network. *Pediatrics*, **107** (1), 14–22.

Horsburgh, M., Lamdin, R. & Williamson, E. (2001) Multi-professional learning: the attitudes of medical, nursing and pharmacy students to shared learning. *Medical Education*, **35**, 876–83.

Howkins, E. & Allison, A. (1997) Shared learning for primary health care teams: a success story. *Nurse Education Today*, **17** (3), 225–31.

Huber, G. & Van de Ven, A. (1995) *Longitudinal Field Research Methods: Studying Processes of Organisational Change*. Sage, Thousand Oaks, Calif.

Hughes, L. & Lucas, J. (1997) An evaluation of problem-based learning in the multi-professional education curriculum for the health professions. *Journal of Interprofessional Care*, **11** (1), 77–88.

Hunter, M. & Love, C. (1996) Total quality management and the reduction of inpatient violence and costs in a forensic psychiatric hospital. *Psychiatric Services*, **47** (7), 751–54.

International Committee of Medical Journal Editors (2003) Uniform requirements for manuscripts. Available from: http://www.icmje.org/index.html (accessed 7 July 2004).

Irvine Doran, D., Baker, R., Murray, M., *et al.* (2002) Achieving clinical improvement: an interdisciplinary initiative. *Health Care Management Review*, **27**, 42–56.

Jackson, P. & McKergow, M. (2002) *The Solutions Focus: the SIMPLE Way to Positive Change.* Nicholas Brealey Publications, London.

Janis, I. (1982) *Groupthink: a Study of Foreign Policy Decisions and Fiascos.* 2nd edn. Houghton Mifflin, Boston, Mass.

Jaques, D. (2000) *Learning in Groups: a Handbook for Improving Groupwork.* 3rd edn. Kogan Page, London.

Juntunen, A. & Heikkinen, E. (2004) Lessons from interprofessional e-learning: piloting a care of the elderly module. *Journal of Interprofessional Care*, **18** (3), 269–78.

Kelly, A. (2004) *The Curriculum: Theory and Practice.* 5th edn. Sage, London.

Ker, J., Mole, L. & Bradley, P. (2003) Early introduction of interprofessional learning: a simulated ward environment. *Medical Teacher*, **37**, 248–55.

Knight, P. (2001) Complexity and curriculum: a process approach to curriculum-making. *Teaching in Higher Education*, **6**, 370–81.

Knowles, M., Holton, E. & Swanson, R. (1998) *The Adult Learner.* 5th edn. Gulf Publishing Company, Houston, Texas.

Kolb, D. (1984) *Experiential Learning.* Prentice Hall, Englewood Cliffs, NJ.

Lalonde, B., Huba, G., Panter, A., *et al.* (2002) Impact of HIV/AIDS education on health care provider practice: results from nine grantees of the special projects of national significance program. *Evaluation and the Health Professions*, **25** (3), 302–320.

Lary, M., Lavigne, S., Muma, S., Jones, S. & Hoeft, H. (1997) Breaking down barriers: multidisciplinary education model. *Journal of Allied Health*, **26**, 63–9.

LaSala, K., Hopper, S., Rissmeyer, D. & Shipe, D. (1997) Rural health care and interdisciplinary education. *Nursing and Health Care Perspectives*, **18** (6), 292–8.

Lave, J. & Wenger, E. (1991) *Situated Learning. Legitimate Peripheral Participation.* University of Cambridge Press, Cambridge.

Leathard, A. (1994) Interprofessional developments in Britain: an overview. In: *Going Interprofessional: Working Together for Health and Welfare* (ed. A. Leathard) Routledge, London.

Lia-Hoagberg, B., Nelson, P. & Chase, R. (1997) An interdisciplinary health team training program for school staff in Minnesota. *Journal of School Health*, **67**, 94–7.

Light, G. & Cox, R. (2001) *Learning and Teaching in Higher Education: the Reflective Professional.* Paul Chapman, London.

Long, S. (1996) Primary health care team workshop: team members' perspectives. *Journal of Advanced Nursing*, **23** (5), 935–41.

Luecht, R., Madson, M., Taugher, M. & Petterson, J. (1990) Assessing perceptions: design and validation of an interdisciplinary education perception scale. *Journal of Allied Health*, **19**, 181–91.

McCoy, S., Cope, K., Joy, S., Baker, R. & Brugler, C. (1997) Interdisciplinary documentation of patient education: how collaboration can effect change. *Rehabilitation Nursing*, **22**, 235–8.

McGill, I. & Beaty, L. (2001) *Action Learning: a Guide for Professional, Management and Educational Development.* Revised 2nd edn. Kogan Page, London.

Mackay, S. (2004) The role perception questionnaire (RPQ): a tool for assessing under-graduate students' perceptions of the role of other professions. *Journal of Interprofessional Care*, **18** (3), 289–302.

Manktelow, J. (2003) Critical path analysis and PERT charts – planning and scheduling more complex projects. Available from: http://www.mindtools.com/critpath.html (accessed 5 July 2004).

Mason, J. (2002) *Qualitative Researching*. 2nd edn. Sage, London.

May, T. (ed.) (2002) *Qualitative Research in Action*. Sage, London.

Mayo, E. (1952) *The Human Problems of an Industrial Civilisation*. 2nd edn. Bailey & Swinfen, Harvard, Mass.

Meads, G. and Ashcroft, J., with Barr, H., Scott, K. & Wild, A. (2005) *The Case for Inter-professional Collaboration*. Blackwell Publishing, Oxford.

Mhaolrúnaigh, S. & Clifford, C. (1998) Parsell, G. & Bligh, J. (1998) Educational principles underpinning successful shared learning. *Medical Teacher*, **20**, 522–9.

Miller, C., Ross, N. & Freeman, M. (1999) *Shared Learning and Clinical Teamwork: New Directions in Education for Multi-professional Practice*. English National Board for Nursing, Midwifery and Health Visiting, London.

Mitchell, B., McCrorie, P. & Sedgwick, P. (2004) Student attitudes towards anatomy teach-ing and learning in a multi-professional context. *Medical Education*, **38**, 737–48.

Morey, J., Simon, R., Jay, G. *et al.* (2002) Error reduction and performance in the emergency department through formal teamwork training: evaluation results of the MedTeams Project. *Health Services Journal*, **37** (6), 1553–81.

Morison, S., Booham, M., Jenkins, J. & Moutray, M. (2003) Facilitating undergraduate interprofessional learning in health-care: comparing classroom and clinical learning for nursing and medical students. *Learning in Health and Social Care*, **2**, 92–104.

Moseley, A. (1997) Teaching Teachers: The East Anglian Interprofessional Practice Teach-ing Programme at the University of East Anglia. *CAIPE Bulletin*, 13, pp. 23–4. London.

National Education Research Forum (2000) *The Impact of Educational Research on Policy and Practice: Subgroup Report*. National Education Research Forum, London. Available from: www.nerf-uk.org/software/impact_report.doc?version = 1 (accessed 5 June 2004).

National Health Service Executive (1993) *Improving Clinical Effectiveness*. Executive Letter EL(93)115. Department of Health, London.

National Health Service Executive (1996) *Achieving Effective Practice: a Clinical Effectiveness and Research Information Pack for Nurses, Midwives and Health Visitors*. NHS Executive, Leeds.

National Health Service Executive (1998) *Promoting Clinical Effectiveness: a Framework for Action In and Through the NHS*. NHS Executive, Leeds. Available from: http://www.dh.gov.uk/assetRoot/04/04/24/62/04042462.pdf (accessed 12 August 2004).

Newell, R. (2001) Writing academic papers: a guide for prospective authors. *Intensive Critical Care Nursing*, **17** (2), 110–16.

Newton, J., Bower, E. & Williams, A. (2004) Research in primary dental care: part VII: writing up your research. *British Dental Journal*, **197**, 121–4.

Nolte, M., Berkery, R., Pizzo, B., *et al.* (1998) Assuring the optimal use of serotonin antagon-ist antiemetics: the process for development and implementation of institutional antie-metic guidelines at Memorial Sloan-Kettering Cancer Center. *Journal of Clinical Oncology*, **16** (2), 771–8.

Oppenheim, A. (1992 & 2000) *Questionnaire Design and Attitudes Measurement*. New edn (1992), Pinter, London. Reissued (2000), Continuum, London.

Øvretveit, J. (1998) *Evaluating Health Initiatives: an Introduction to Evaluation of Health Treatments, Services, Policies and Organisational Initiatives.* Open University Press, Buckingham.

Parlett, M. (1981) Illuminative evaluation. In: *Human Inquiry* (eds P. Reason & J. Rowan), pp. 219–26. John Wiley & Sons, London.

Parsell, G. & Bligh, J. (1999) The development of a questionnaire to assess the readiness of health care students for interprofessional learning (RIPLS). *Medical Education,* **33,** 95–100.

Patton, M. (2002) *Qualitative Research and Evaluation Methods.* 3rd edn. Sage, London.

Pawson, R. & Tilly, N. (1997) *Realistic Evaluation.* Sage, London.

Perkins, J. & Tryssenaar, J. (1994) Making interdisciplinary education effective for rehabilitation students. *Journal of Allied Health,* **23** (3), 133–41.

Pirrie, A., Wilson, V., Harden, R. & Elsegood, J. (1998) AMEE Guide No. 12: multi-professional education: part II: promoting cohesive practice in health care. *Medical Teacher,* **20,** 409–416.

Pope, C. & Mays, N. (eds) (1999) *Qualitative Research in Health Care.* Revised edn, British Medical Journal *Books, London.*

Posner, G. (2003) *Analysing the Curriculum.* McGraw-Hill, Boston.

Poulton, B. & West, M. (1993) Effective multidisciplinary teamwork in primary health care. *Journal of Advanced Nursing,* **18,** 918–25.

Poulton, B. & West, M. (1994) Primary health care team effectiveness: developing a constituency approach. *Health and Social Care in the Community,* **2,** 77–84.

Poulton, B. & West, M. (1999) The determinants of effectiveness in primary health care teams. *Journal of Interprofessional Care,* **13,** 7–18.

Price, J., Ekleberry, A., Grover, A., *et al.* (1999) Evaluation of clinical practice guidelines on outcome of infection in patients in the surgical intensive care unit. *Critical Medical Care,* **27** (10), 2118–24.

Pryce, A. & Reeves, S. (1997) *An Evaluation of the Effectiveness of Multidisciplinary Education for Medical, Dental and Nursing students: a Case Study.* City University, London. Available from: http://www.city.ac.uk/barts/research/reports/pdf/reeves_s/mem.pdf (accessed 20 July 2004).

Quality Assurance Agency for Higher Education (2001) *Benchmarking Academic and Practitioner Standards in Health Care Subjects/Professions.* Quality Assurance Agency for Higher Education, Gloucester.

Quality Assurance Agency for Higher Education (2002a) *Benchmarking Standards in Biomedical Science.* Quality Assurance Agency for Higher Education, Gloucester. Available from: http://www.qaa.ac.uk/crntwork/benchmark/phase2/biomedsci.pdf (accessed 15 August 2004).

Quality Assurance Agency for Higher Education (2002b) *Benchmarking Standards in Dentistry.* Quality Assurance Agency for Higher Education, Gloucester. Available from: www.qaa.ac.uk/crntwork/benchmark/phase2/Dentistry.pdf (accessed 15 August 2004).

Quality Assurance Agency for Higher Education (2002c) *Benchmarking Standards in Health Studies.* Quality Assurance Agency for Higher Education, Gloucester. Available from: www.qaa.ac.uk/crntwork/benchmark/phase2/healthstudies.pdf (accessed 15 August 2004).

Quality Assurance Agency for Higher Education (2002d) *Benchmarking Standards in Medicine.* Quality Assurance Agency for Higher Education, Gloucester. Available from: http://www.qaa.ac.uk/crntwork/benchmark/phase2/medicine.pdf (accessed 15 August 2004).

Quality Assurance Agency for Higher Education (2002e) *Benchmarking Standards in Optometry.* Quality Assurance Agency for Higher Education, Gloucester. Available from: www.qaa.ac.uk/crntwork/benchmark/phase2/optometry.pdf (accessed 15 August 2004).

Quality Assurance Agency for Higher Education (2002f) *Benchmarking Standards in Pharmacy.* Quality Assurance Agency for Higher Education, Gloucester. Available from: www.qaa.ac.uk/crntwork/benchmark/phase2/pharmacy.pdf (accessed 15 August 2004).

Quality Assurance Agency for Higher Education (2002g) *Benchmarking Standards in Social Policy and Administration and Social Work.* Quality Assurance Agency for Higher Education, Gloucester. Available from: http://www.qaa.ac.uk/crntwork/benchmark/social-work.pdf (accessed 15 August 2004).

Quinn, F. M. (1994) The demise of the curriculum. In: *Health Care Education: the Challenge of the Market Place* (eds T. Humphreys & F.M. Quinn) Nelson Thornes, Cheltenham.

Ramsden, P. (2003) *Learning to Teach in Higher Education.* 2nd edn. Routledge, London.

Reason, P. & Bradbury, H. (2000) *The Handbook of Action Research: Participative Inquiry and Practice.* Sage, London.

Reeves, S. (2000) Community-based interprofessional education for medical, nursing and dental students. *Health and Social Care in the Community.* **8** (4), 269–76.

Reeves, S. (2005) Developing and delivering practice-based interprofessional education: successes and challenges. Unpublished Ph.D. Thesis, City University, London.

Reeves, S., Freeth, D., Nicol, M. & Wood, D. (2000) A joint learning venture between new nurses and junior doctors. *Nursing Times,* **96** (38), 39–40.

Richardson, B. & Cooper, N. (2003) Developing a virtual interdisciplinary research community in higher education. *Journal of Interprofessional Care,* **17**, 173–82.

Roberts, C., Howe, A., Winterburn, S. & Fox, N. (2000) Not so easy as it sounds: a qualitative study of a shared learning project between medical and nursing undergraduate students. *Medical Teacher,* **22**, 386–7.

Robson, C. (2002) *Real World Research: a Resource for Social Scientists and Practitioner Researchers.* 2nd edn. Blackwell Publishing, Oxford.

Rossi, P., Lipsey, M. & Freeman, H. (2004) *Evaluation: a Systematic Approach.* 7th edn. Sage, Newbury Park, California.

Rossi, P., Wright, J. & Anderson, A. (eds) (1985) *Handbook of Survey Research.* Academic Press, NY.

Rowntree, D. (1991) *Statistics without Tears.* Penguin, London.

Rubenstein, L.V., Parker, L.E., Meredith, L.S., *et al.* (2002) Understanding team-based quality improvement for depression in primary care. *Health Services Research,* **37** (4), 1009–1029.

Sackett, D., Richardson, W., Rosenberg, W. & Haynes, R. (1997) *Evidence-based Medicine: How to Practice and Teach EBM.* Churchill Livingstone, New York.

Salmon, G. (2004) *E-moderating: the Key to Teaching and Learning Online.* 2nd edn. Routledge, London.

Savin-Baden, M. (2003) *Facilitating Problem-based Learning: Illuminating Perspectives.* SRHE and Open University Press, Maidenhead.

Schreiber, M., Holcomb, J., Conaway, C., Campbell, K., Wall, M. & Mattox, K. (2002) Military trauma training performed in a civilian trauma center. *Journal of Surgical Research,* **104** (1), 8–14.

Schön, D. (1987) *Educating the Reflective Practitioner: Toward a New Design for Teaching and Learning in the Professions*. Jossey-Bass, San Francisco.

Scott, D. (ed.) (2001) *Curriculum and Assessment (International Perspectives on Curriculum Studies)*. Ablex Publishing, London.

Shafer, M.A., Tebb, K.P., Pantell, R.M., *et al.* (2002) Effect of a clinical practice improvement intervention on chlamydial screening among adolescent girls. *Journal of American Medical Association*, **288** (22), 2846–52.

Silverman, D. (2000) *Doing Qualitative Research: A Practical Handbook*. Sage, London.

Singh, N., Wechsler, H., Curtis, J., Sabaawi, M., Myers, R. & Singh, S. (2002) Effects of role-play and mindfulness training on enhancing the family friendliness of the admissions treatment team processes *Journal of Emotional and Behavioural Disorders*, **10** (2), 90–98.

Smith, H., Armstrong, M. & Brown, S. (1999) *Benchmarking and Threshold Standards in Higher Education*. Kogan Page, London.

Sommer, S., Silagy, C. & Rose, A. (1992) The teaching of multidisciplinary care. *Medical Journal of Australia*, **157**, 31–7.

Stagnaro-Green, A. (2004) Applying adult learning principles to medical education in the United States. *Medical Teacher*, **26** (1), 79–85.

Stake, R. (1975) *Evaluating the Arts in Education: a Responsive Approach*. Merrill, Columbus, Ohio.

Stephenson, J. & Yorke, M. (eds) (1998) *Capability and Quality in Higher Education*. Kogan Page, London.

Stone, J. A. M., Haas, B. A., Harmer-Beem, M. J. & Baker, D. L. (2004) Utilisation of research methodology in designing an interdisciplinary course in ethics. *Journal of Interprofessional Care*, **18** (1), 55–62.

Sully, P. (2002) Commitment to partnership: interdisciplinary initiatives in developing expert practice in the care of survivors of violence. *Nurse Education in Practice*, **2**, 92–8.

Swage, T. (2003) *Clinical Governance in Health Care Practice*. 2nd edn. Butterworth-Heinemann, Oxford.

Tashakkori, A. & Teddlie, C. (2002) *Handbook of Mixed Methods in Social and Behavioural Research*. Sage, London.

Thackwray, B. (1997) *Effective Evaluation of Training and Development in Higher Education*. Taylor and Francis, London.

Thomas, M. (1995) Learning to be a better team-player: initiatives in continuing education in primary health care. In: *Interprofessional Relations in Health Care* (eds K. Soothill, L. Mackay & C. Webb) pp. 194–215. Edward Arnold, London.

Thompson, C., Kinmonth, A., Stevens, L., *et al.* (2000) Effects of a clinical-practice guideline and practice-based education on detection and outcome of depression in primary care: Hampshire Depression Project randomised controlled trial. *The Lancet*, **355** (9199), 185–91.

Tuckman, B. (1965) Developmental sequence in small groups. *Psychological Bulletin*, **63**, 384–99.

Tuckman, B. & Jensen, M. (1977) Stages of small group development revisited. *Group and Organisational Studies*, **2**, 419–27.

WHO (1998) *Health for all in the Twenty-first Century*. World Health Organization, Geneva.

van der Horst, M., Turpie, I., Nelson, W., *et al.* (1995) St Joseph's Community Health Centre model of community-based interdisciplinary health care team. *Health and Social Care in the Community*, **3**, 33–42.

van Staa A.L., Visser, A. & van der Zouwe, N. (2000) Caring for caregivers: experiences and evaluation of initiatives for a palliative care team. *Patient Education and Counselling*, **41** (1), 93–105.

Williams, G. & Laungani, P. (1999) Analysis of teamwork in an NHS community trust: an empirical study. *Journal of Interprofessional Care*, **13**, 19–28.

Yin, R. (2003) *Case Study Research: Design and Methods*. 3rd edn. Sage, London.

Zwarenstein, M., Reeves, S., Barr, H., Hammick, M., Koppel, I. & Atkins, J. (2001) Interprofessional education: effects on professional practice and health care outcomes (Cochrane Review) http://www.update-software.com/ccweb/cochrane/revabstr/ab002213.htm

Index